Health-Related Fitness
for Grades 1 and 2

Chris Hopper, PhD
Humboldt State University

Bruce Fisher
Fortuna Elementary School

Kathy D. Munoz, EdD
Humboldt State University

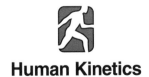

Human Kinetics

We dedicate this book to our families—

Renee, Molly, Ian, and Andrew;

Rich, Heather, Wesley, and Ryan;

Mindi and Jenny.

Library of Congress Cataloging-in-Publication Data

Hopper, Christopher A., 1952–
    Health-related fitness for grades 1 and 2 / Chris Hopper, Bruce
Fisher, Kathy D. Munoz.
      p.   cm.
    Includes index.
    ISBN 0-87322-498-1
    1. Physical fitness for children.   2. Exercise for children.
3. Children—Health and hygiene.   I. Fisher, Bruce, 1949– .
II. Munoz, Kathy, 1951– .   III. Title.
GV443.H645   1997
613.7'042—dc20   96-12408
                              CIP

ISBN: 0-87322-498-1

Acquisitions Editor: Scott Wikgren; **Developmental Editor:** Nanette Smith; **Assistant Editor:** Henry Woolsey; **Editorial Assistant:** Coree Schutter; **Copyeditors:** Denelle Eknes, Julia Anderson; **Indexer:** Barbara E. Cohen; **Typesetting and Layout:** Impressions Book and Journal Services, Inc.; **Graphic Designer:** Judy Henderson; **Cover Designer:** Jack Davis; **Illustrators:** Mary Yemma Long, Nicole Barbuto, Craig Ronto, Dianna Porter; **Printer:** Versa Press

Printed in the United States of America

10 9 8 7 6 5 4 3 2 1

Human Kinetics
Web site: http://www.humankinetics.com/

United States: Human Kinetics
P.O. Box 5076, Champaign, IL 61825-5076
1-800-747-4457
e-mail: humank@hkusa.com

Canada: Human Kinetics
Box 24040, Windsor, ON N8Y 4Y9
1-800-465-7301 (in Canada only)
e-mail: humank@hkcanada.com

Europe: Human Kinetics
P.O. Box IW14, Leeds LS16 6TR, United Kingdom
(44) 1132 781708
e-mail: humank@hkeurope.com

Australia: Human Kinetics
57A Price Avenue, Lower Mitcham, South Australia 5062
(08) 277 1555
e-mail: humank@hkaustralia.com

New Zealand: Human Kinetics
P.O. Box 105-231, Auckland 1
(09) 523 3462
e-mail: humank@hknewz.com

Contents

Appendixes   105

Preface

In recent years the following headlines have appeared in the media:

Young Adults More Fat Than Fit, Study Finds

Lorem ipsum dolor sit amet, consectetuer adipiscing elit, euismod tincidunt magna aliquam enim ad minim erci tation ulla nisl ut aliquip Duis autem vel drerit in vulput sequat, vel illum facilisis at vero

Lorem ipsum dolor sit amet, consectetuer

Any Exercise is Good Exercise: Experts say even a little moderate activity goes a long way

Lorem ipsum dolor sit amet, consectetuer adipiscing elit, sed diam nonummy nibh euismod tincidunt ut laoreet dolore magna aliquam erat volutpat. Ut wisi enim ad minim quis nostrud exerci tation ullamcorper suscipit lobortis nisl ut aliquip ex ea commodo consequat. Duis autem vel eum iure dolor in hendrerit in vulputate velit

Lorem ipsum dolor sit amet, consectetuer adipiscing elit, sed diam nonummy nibh euismod tincidunt ut laoreet dolore magna aliquam erat volutpat. Ut wisi enim ad minim veniam, quis nostrud exerci tation ullamcorper suscipit lobortis nisl ut aliquip ex ea commodo consequat. Duis autem vel eum iriure dolor in hendrerit in vulputate velit

FITNESS: Study Finds Big Slip

Lorem ipsum dolor sit amet, consectetuer adipiscing elit, sed diam nonummy nibh euismod tincidunt ut laoreet dolore

lore te feugait nulla facilisi. tempor cum soluta nobis elei congue nihil imperdiet domi erat facer possim a m dolor sit amet, elit, sed diam non incidunt ut lao uam e nim ve ullamc ip ex vel eu putate vero

Kids Confused On Health, Survey Finds

Lorem ipsum dolor sit amet, consectetuer   facilisis at vero eros et accumsan et justo

Young People's Health Declining, Report Says

Lorem ipsum dolor sit amet, consectetuer adipiscing elit, sed diam nonummy nibh euismod tincidunt ut laoreet dolore magna aliquam erat volutpat. Ut wisi enim ad minim veniam, quis nostrud exerci tation ullamcorper suscipit lobortis nisl ut aliquip ex ea commodo consequat. Duis autem vel eum iriure dolor in hendrerit in vulputate velit esse molestie consequat, vel illum dolore eu feug accumsan et justo odio dignissim qui b delenit augue duis dolore te feugait nulla amet, consectetuer adipiscing elit, sed tincidunt ut laoreet dolore magna aliqu ad minim veniam, quis nostrud exerci ta tis nisl ut aliquip ex ea commodo conseq Duis autem vel eum iriure dolor in hend lestie consequat, vel illum dolore eu feug accumsan et justo odio dignissim qui b delenit augue duis dolore te feugait nulla soluta nobis eleifend option congue nih mazim placerat facer possim assum.

FAT: Even Moderate Weight Gains Are Risky

Lorem ipsum dolor sit amet, consectetuer   amet, consectetuer adipiscing elit, sed n nonummy nibh euismod tincidunt at. Ut wisi enim ad minim veniam, s nostrud exerci tation ullamcorper cipit lobortis nisl ut aliquip ex ea com do consequat. s autem vel eum iriure dolor in hen quat, vel illum dolore eu feugiat nulla lisis at vero eros et accumsan et justo zzril delenit augue duis dolore te feu nulla facilisi. Nam liber tempor cum

Vigorous Exercise Adds On Years, Study Says

Lorem ipsum dolor sit amet, consectetuer adipiscing elit, sed diam nonummy nibh euismod tincidunt ut laoreet dolore magna aliquam erat volutpat. Ut wisi enim ad minim veniam, quis nostrud exerci tation ullamcorper suscipit lobortis nisl ut aliquip ex ea commodo consequat. Duis autem vel eum iriure dolor in hendrerit in vulputate velit esse molestie con-

sequat, vel illum dolore eu feugiat nulla facilisis at vero eros et accumsan et justo odio dignissim qui blandit praesent luptatum zzril delenit augue duis dolore te feugait nulla facilisi. Lorem ipsum dolor sit amet, consectetuer adipiscing elit, sed diam nonummy nibh euismod tincidunt ut laoreet dolore magna aliquam erat volutpat. Ut wisi enim ad minim veniam,

Overall, considerable evidence suggests that the cardiovascular health of children is at risk.

As a teacher, you're as concerned about the cardiovascular health of kids as are parents and medical professionals. You know if kids develop healthy habits when they're in elementary school, chances are they'll become healthy adolescents and adults. With the lively and seasoned activities and lessons in this book, you can incorporate sound cardiovascular wellness into your classroom. Whether you are an elementary school teacher developing physical education lessons or a physical education specialist, you'll find this an invaluable and complete guide to promoting cardiovascular health through daily lessons.

Chris Hopper and Kathy Munoz teach in the Department of Health and Physical Education at Humboldt State University and have worked extensively with teachers in Northern California to improve instruction in physical education and nutrition. Their work has been published in research journals such as *Research Quarterly for Exercise and Sport* and teacher journals such as *Learning*. Bruce Fisher was California Teacher of the Year in 1991 and serves as a consultant for health education to the California Department of Education. Bruce is recognized by his colleagues as an innovative teacher. All three authors have tested the lessons in this book, which represents a decade of professional work.

The authors designed this book to enhance existing physical education programs and to be a comprehensive resource for teachers who want to spice up their teaching with fun-filled, exciting learning activities. This book includes physical education activity lessons that emphasize children enjoying movement.

The fitness and nutrition information includes cardiovascular fitness, strength, endurance, flexibility, fat, carbohydrates, water, sodium, and heart-healthy eating. The goal of the book is to communicate the need for a lifelong commitment to health and physical fitness, using cardiovascular exercise and diet. The goal for you in using the book is to change the attitudes and behaviors of children so they embrace this commitment to health and fitness.

The book emphasizes ready-to-go activities and materials teachers can easily use. The book has a user friendly approach with illustrations, pages to copy, and lesson outlines. We recognize that classroom teachers are extremely busy. The format and design eliminate extra work.

Teachers can meet multiple teaching objectives by using this curriculum. Unique features include cross-curriculum activities, meaningful homework, and cooperative learning activities. In addition, while children are studying fitness and nutrition, they'll be developing research techniques (surveys), critical thinking skills (comparing foods), science concepts (e.g., how the heart works), language arts (e.g., food label analysis), and mathematical applications (e.g., counting pulse rates).

The program covers nine weeks of fitness and nutrition education and activities related to cardiovascular health. Each week includes five 30-minute lessons, with one concept development and discussion lesson, three physical education activity lessons, and one nutrition concept lesson. The lessons are divided into the following sections:

Heart Facts (1 week)

What's in a Workout? (1 week)

Fitness Components (1 week)

Risk Factors (1 week)

Aerobic Fitness concepts (2 weeks)

Flexibility Fitness concepts (1 week)

Strength Fitness concepts (1 week)

Healthy Lifestyle (1 week)

This book is the first in a series of three books designed to enhance the cardiovascular health of children. Be sure to review *Health-Related Fitness for Grades 3 and 4* and *Health-Related Fitness for Grades 5 and 6*.

Acknowledgments

We thank the following teachers for help in pilot testing: Linda Provancha, Fred Johansen, Steve Wartburg, and Linda Buron.

We also thank Tami Jaegel for researching information, and Ira Samuels and Mike Mullane for their advice.

We thank Tricia Gill, Elissa Fisher, and Linda Baxter for typing the manuscript.

Introduction to Curriculum

Before starting the curriculum, include an introduction to the lessons and explain the lesson objectives and purposes.

Objectives

1. To teach the basic elements of a healthy cardiovascular system (lungs, heart, and blood vessels)
2. To introduce important fitness and nutrition concepts for a healthy heart
3. To teach children how to plan and develop their own exercise programs

Teaching Strategies

- Use laminated task cards with names of specific exercises and activities that you can use as a resource. Use the exercises in chapter 13 to develop cards.
- Stress that children don't have heart attacks. Children develop lifestyle habits that put them at risk for heart disease later in life.
- Avoid simply repeating jumping jacks, windmills, and so forth, with no purpose. Put them into a game or activity.
- Don't use running laps or other exercises as a punishment for bad behavior.
- Use writing projects about exercise and nutrition to improve language arts.
- Avoid elimination activities.

Cross-Curricular Themes

We have identified the following cross-curricular areas in the lessons:

- Health

- Visual and Performing Arts

- Science

- Mathematics

- Language Arts

Nutrition Education

In nutrition education students gain the knowledge, skills, and motivation they need to make wise food choices. They learn that healthy foods are intimately connected with physical, mental, emotional, and social health. Also, energy, self-image, and physical fitness are related to heart-healthy nutrition. A comprehensive nutrition education program integrates nutrition lessons with the core curriculum. Lessons in this book include classroom activities for food tasting, preparation, and menu planning.

Home Activities

Home activities provide a connection between the home and the school, strengthening the school-family relationship. Parents as care providers can dramatically influence eating habits and physical activity levels. They buy and prepare food for children and determine restaurant choices. In addition, parents help their children make significant choices regarding exercise. Parents can register their children for sport and activity programs and tell their children to turn off the television. In overall lifestyle, parents serve as gatekeepers, and children are unlikely to change their lifestyles without the support of their parents.

A Lesson a Day for Nine Weeks

We organized the curriculum to provide a lesson a day for nine weeks. This concentrated approach will give students the knowledge and skills to make significant lifestyle changes. The curriculum is sequential, with basic knowledge introduced, then applied to cardiovascular health.

Discussion Lessons

Discussion lessons are an essential component of the curriculum and allow students to reflect on important concepts about physical fitness and nutrition. These lessons develop the skills and knowledge of physical fitness and nutrition that are the foundation of a healthy lifestyle.

Warming Up and Cooling Down

Each lesson should start with a warm-up and finish with a cool-down.

Warm-Up = Light Activity + Stretching

A warm-up before exercise prepares your body for activity and avoids "jump starting" the body. Warm-ups stretch muscles and help prevent muscle soreness and injury. In addition, warm-ups prepare the heart for more vigorous activity and avoid adding stress.

Exercise specialists recommend completing light activity first, such as jogging, followed by gentle static stretching (see basic warm-up and cool-down stretches on pages 89–92). Remember not to bounce when stretching. A listing of warm-up activities is found on pages 89–90. Most of these include jogging or light running.

Although children rarely stretch before going out to recess or playing vigorous activities, stretching is an investment for the future. Joints that are flexible in childhood will gradually lose mobility with age, leading to a reduced range of movement. Developing a lifetime habit of stretching before exercise can pay dividends now and later.

Cool-Down = Less Vigorous Activity + Stretching

The cool-down is an essential part of any exercise session. It is just as important as the warm-up. A cool-down should last about five minutes and allow your body to gently recover after vigorous exercise. An abrupt end to exercise sends your blood pressure fluctuating like a yo-yo. This leads to slow removal of waste products. Light activity and stretching continue the pumping action of muscles on veins, helping the circulation remove wastes. Static stretching may help reduce delayed soreness or muscle pain the day after exercise. Cool-down activities are found on pages 91–92.

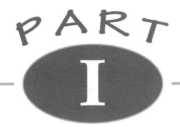

Weekly Lessons

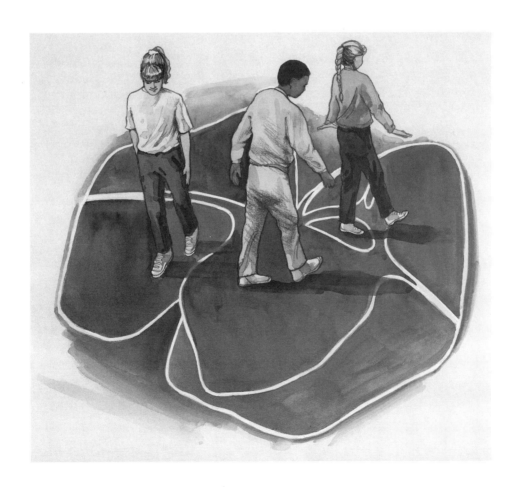

Week 1: Heart Facts

The lessons emphasize understanding the location, structure, and function of the heart. The physical activity lessons reinforce specific concepts about the heart, arteries, and veins. In nutrition, children learn to place foods in categories depending on plant or animal origin.

Lesson 1

Heart Facts

WEEK 1

Goals

- To identify the size and location of the heart
- To introduce the function of the heart

Key Concepts

The heart is about the size of a fist and its job is to pump blood to the body. The heart is located in the center of the chest. The heart pumps all the time without taking a rest. It pumps blood to all parts of the body. The heart is a muscle with a hollow inside consisting of four chambers.

Materials

1. Butcher paper
2. Felt-tip pens
3. Picture of heart (figure 1.1)
4. Sample body outline with heart in proper place (make before lesson)
5. Red construction paper
6. Scissors

Activity: Heart Facts

- Students work in pairs and trace a body outline of each other while lying on a piece of butcher paper.
- Keep the outline of each child to use in later lessons.
- Use the outline to attach a picture of the heart in the body in the correct location. Ask students to draw on a piece of 8 × 11 red construction paper what they think their heart looks like. Tell them it is the size of a fist to get them started.
- After they have attempted a drawing, show them a picture of the heart (figure 1.1) and ask them to redraw their heart.

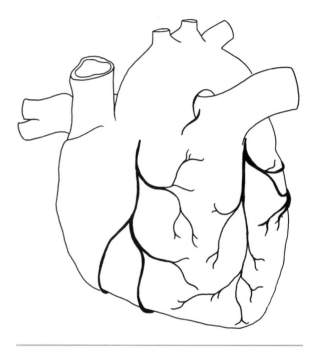

Fig. 1.1   The child's heart

- Have students feel the beat of their own hearts. They can now correctly place their heart on the body outline.

Teaching Tips

If students are unable to feel their heartbeats, do 20 to 30 seconds of exercise (jogging in place). Demonstrate how to draw the outline. Pair children with members of the same gender and help them with their outlines. Add details such as facial features to personalize outlines. Students could work with cross-age tutors for more accurate drawings and cutouts. Save body outlines for lesson 36.

WEEK 1

Lesson 2

Follow the Red and Blue Road

Goals

- To introduce the concept that blood travels in tubes within the body
- To understand that red blood travels in the arteries and blue blood in the veins
- To improve cardiovascular endurance

Key Concepts

Arteries and veins are the major blood vessels of the vascular system. Arteries carry blood away from the heart and veins carry blood back to the heart from body organs and body parts.

Materials

1. Playground chalk, jump ropes, cones, or other markers
2. Twenty (10 red and 10 blue) cones to represent arteries and veins
3. Red and blue construction paper (if necessary)

Warm-Up: 5 Minutes

Select stretching and warm-up activities.

Activity: Follow the Red and Blue Road

- Using playground chalk, jump ropes, or cones, mark areas representing the head, two arms, two legs, and heart (see figure 1.2). A large playing area (50 × 50 yards) is desirable, although you can use a smaller area.
- Join the heart with the body parts using two lines of cones, one being arteries, the other being veins.
- Use red cones for arteries and blue cones for veins, or indicate red and blue pathways by

attaching a piece of construction paper to cones.
- Students start in the heart and act as the blood. On the command "arteries," students jog to the arms, legs, or head along the arteries (red path).
- Students wait in the periphery of the body until all have arrived. On the command "veins," students jog back to the heart along the blue line of cones representing veins.

Cool-Down: 5 Minutes

Select stretching and cool-down activities.

Teaching Tips

Encourage continuous movement and explain that blood in the body keeps flowing without taking a rest. Allow children to walk if necessary. You can use a drum or tambourine to simulate the heartbeat. The teacher can lead the movement to demonstrate the blood flow pattern; then let children take turns leading. Divide class into squads of five or six students. Children can visit each body part in turn. Vary the movement pattern and include hopping, skipping, and galloping. Students with physical disabilities can walk rather than run with their squad. You can pair students with attention problems with a buddy who provides leadership.

As an additional activity, children sit in a circle and hold hands. A box of foam balls represents the heart. The first person takes a ball out of the box and passes it around the circle. When the ball reaches the last person, they replace it in the box. Then pass more balls around the circle. This represents a blood flow pattern. The teacher can call out an activity and children can adjust rate of blood flow accordingly, for example, sleeping (slow) and running (fast).

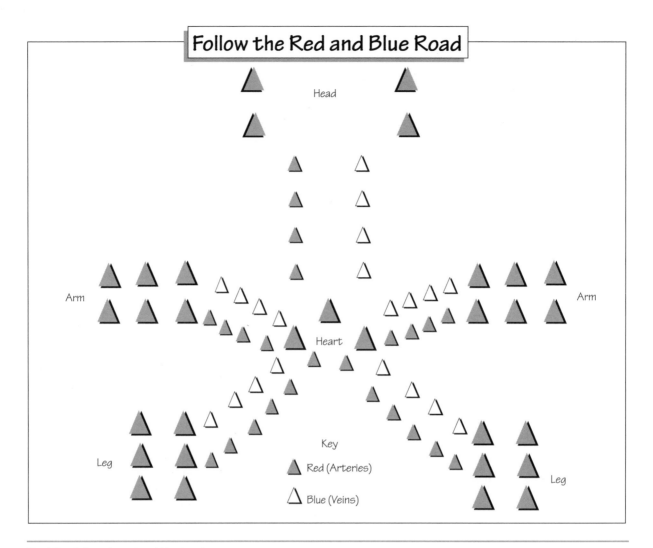

Fig. 1.2   Follow the red and blue road

WEEK 1

Lesson 3

Aerobic Animals

Goals

- To demonstrate a difference between animal and human hearts
- To improve cardiovascular endurance

Key Concepts

The rate at which the heart beats varies widely in animals. In humans the rate varies between 50 and 100 beats per minute. Heart rates in animals depend on the size of the animal and the functioning they need for survival. Generally, smaller animals have faster heart rates. Animals that need to move quickly for survival have higher heart rates.

Materials

1. Playground chalk, jump ropes, cones, or other markers
2. Drum (optional)
3. Red and blue cones

Warm-Up: 5 Minutes

Select stretching and warm-up activities.

Activity: Aerobic Animals

- Using chalk, jump ropes, or cones, mark areas representing the head, two arms, two legs, and the heart.
- Students start in the heart and act as blood moving through the body. The blood moves to the head, arms, or legs, and back to the heart.
- Students can move according to the rate at which the heart beats in the designated animal. Vary the animal selected by calling out the names of different animals.
- The children can perform movements imitating animal locomotion if using an indoor facility.

- Use the following guide for movement speed:

  Mouse 650 beats per minute (sprint)
  Cat 110 beats per minute (jog)
  Dog 80 beats per minute (skip)
  Child 80 beats per minute (skip)
  Tiger 40 beats per minute (walk)
  Tortoise 30 beats per minute (slow motion)

Cool-Down: 5 Minutes

Select stretching and cool-down activities.

Teaching Tips

You can use a drum to simulate the heartbeat. Emphasize using arms in opposition to legs in all forms of movement (sprint, jog, skip, walk). Encourage children to keep moving.

WEEK 1

Lesson 4
A Piece of My Heart

Goals

- To understand that the heart consists of four chambers
- To improve cardiovascular endurance

Key Concepts

The heart has four chambers (or rooms), left and right auricles and left and right ventricles. The top chambers on each side of the heart are the auricles and the bottom chambers are the ventricles. Blood enters the heart through the auricles and leaves through the ventricles.

Materials

1. Draw the picture of the heart with four chambers (see figure 1.3). Cut heart into four chambers. Repeat on different colored paper and laminate. Make enough hearts so each child has a piece of a puzzle. On the back of each puzzle piece write an exercise task, such as 10 jumping jacks, 5 side leg raises, or 6 mountain climbers.
2. Four cones

Warm-Up: 5 Minutes

Select stretching and warm-up activities.

Activity: A Piece of My Heart

- Mark out a square (40 × 40 yards) with four cones. Students jog around the cones.
- Hand out one puzzle piece to students as they jog by.
- When all students have a puzzle piece, they stop jogging and attempt to match their puzzle piece with other pieces of the same color.
- Students solve the puzzle, which is the four chambers of the heart.
- After completing the puzzle, the children complete the exercise on each puzzle piece as a group (see exercises in chapter 13.)

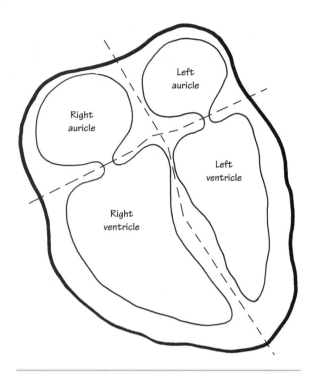

Fig. 1.3 *The four chambers of the heart*

Cool-Down: 5 Minutes

Select stretching and cool-down activities.

Teaching Tips

Label each piece of the puzzle (right and left auricle and ventricle) so children know which piece they have. Vary the way and direction in which children move around the square, including jogging, skipping, walking, sideways shuffle, and running backward.

For students with physical disabilities who are unable to move as fast as other students, allow them to pick up a piece of the heart after completing one length of the square.

WEEK 1

Lesson 5

What's to Eat?

Goals

- To identify foods that come from plants and animals
- To classify different foods according to their origin (plant versus animal)

Key Concepts

We eat food to provide energy to live and grow. We also eat when we feel hungry and because we enjoy eating. The food we choose to eat comes from a variety of plant and animal sources. Students will learn that foods contain different components, namely fat, protein, and carbohydrates, which can be classified as positive (+) or negative (−). These features are referred to as attributes and reflect what foods have in common.

Materials

1. Pictures of the following foods placed on cards: carrots, eggs, rice, butter, oatmeal, sour cream, bananas, fish, oranges, french bread, cereal, milk, broccoli, cheese, bacon, apples, corn, hamburger, and pork chops
2. One yard of string or yarn for each group
3. For the group activity, additional cards with pictures of individual foods to equal 10 cards per group
4. Handout 1.1 Week 1, Family Activity: Favorites Survey (one per student)

Activity: What's to Eat?

- On the board, write a (+) and a (−) with the words carrots under the (+) and eggs under the (–) along with the corresponding picture cards.

(+)	(–)
Carrots	Eggs

- Then ask the students the following:
  "Look at these two pictures of food. How are these foods alike and how are they different? Carrots have the attributes of our positive category. Eggs do not." (Be sure to accept and acknowledge all reasonable responses.)
- Then place the next two picture cards with words on the board beneath the first two:

Rice	Butter

- Say: "Now examine this pair. Rice has the attributes we are concerned with. Butter does not. What do carrots and rice have in common that eggs and butter do not?"
- Ask the students to work in small groups during this phase of the exercise. Present two more food pictures (positive examples are foods that come from plants and negative examples are from animals). Ask the students to compare and contrast them, trying to discover what the positive examples have in common that they do not share with negative examples.

Oatmeal	Sour cream

- "Now what do you see? Discuss what you think are the attributes that the positive foods have in common. How are they different from foods I have identified as negative?"
- After a few seconds place the next two pictures and words on the board:

Bananas	Fish

"Did any of you have to change your ideas?" Then put on the board the following pictures:

Broccoli	Cheddar cheese
Cheerios or cereal	Bacon
Corn	Hamburger
French bread	Pork chops
Apples	Whole milk

Ask again, "Did any of you have to change your ideas?"
- Then say, "Oranges. Based on your thinking, is this positive or negative?" Continue providing one picture or word examples and asking them to identify if they are positive or negative. If they can identify them correctly, ask them to share their hypotheses. Confirm their hypotheses and relate the essential attributes of the positive examples. Ask the students to come up with a few of their own examples.
- Assign groups for the next activity. Provide each group with a string to form a circle and at least 10 pictures of different foods, such as fruits, vegetables, meat, bread, and so forth. Ask them to look for positive and negative examples for each food. Then place the pictures inside the "attribute circle" or string if it is positive (a plant food) or outside the circle if it is negative (an animal food).
- Discuss their findings with the class.
- Have the students exchange cards and instruct each group to create an attribute circle. Instruct each group to place plant foods inside the circle and animal foods outside the circle. After the attribute circle is finished, rotate groups and see if they agree with the results. If they disagree, change the cards. Discuss changes after each rotation.

Teaching Tips

Before this lesson, practice attributing and categorizing with students using examples such as hair color, types of clothing, and height.

The results of handout 1.1, Favorites Survey, could be presented individually by students as part of sharing. Children can report to the class on their survey results.

Several children can be invited to share and the class can keep a tally of favorite activities and foods. You can use this information later in the curriculum, for example, in lesson 21 when children examine different types of activities.

Handout 1.1   Week 1, Family Activity: Favorites Survey

Complete this questionnaire with your family. Parents can help write the answers.

1. List the favorite activity or sport and food of each family member.

Family member   Activity or sport   Food

_____

_____

_____

_____

2. What are the activities that your family participates in together?

3. Do you and your family members do something active every day?

Yes _____

No _____

If not every day, how often each week?

4. What's your favorite breakfast food?

Time: 15 minutes

Please return by _____.

Week 2: What's in a Workout?

The lessons introduce students to the three major phases of a workout. Lessons provide examples of workouts. Students learn about the varying amounts of fat in milk.

Lesson 6

5-20-5

WEEK 2

Goals

- To understand the major components of a workout
- To emphasize the importance of a warm-up and cool-down

Key Concepts

"Every person should accumulate 30 minutes or more of moderate-intensity physical activity over the course of most days of the week." This is a joint recommendation of the U.S. Centers for Disease Control, the American College of Sports Medicine, and the President's Council on Physical Fitness and Sports.

Materials

1. Paper and art supplies for each group
2. Moveable clock face

Activity: 5-20-5

Discuss with your class the three phases of a workout.

a. 5-minute warm-up

A warm-up before exercise helps prepare your body for activity. Warm-ups stretch muscles and help prevent muscle soreness and injury. In addition, warm-ups prepare the heart for more vigorous activity and avoid putting undue stress on the heart.

Start with gentle static stretching. Remember not to bounce when stretching. Then, at a slow speed, do some specific exercises, such as jogging. Gradually increase the pace of your warm-up until you are sweating. Model with class before moving to the next component. Chapter 11 provides warm-up activities.

b. 20-minute workout

Plan the workout section so it includes 20 minutes of continuous activity. Activities that are continuous and use large muscle groups of the body are ideal. Select activities that develop strength and endurance, such as sit-ups and push-ups, along with games and drills that involve running or jogging. Model with the class.

c. 5-minute cool-down

The cool-down is an important part of any exercise session and just as essential as the warm-up. A cool-down should last five minutes and allow your body to gently return to normal. Stopping an activity abruptly sends your blood pressure bouncing like a yo-yo and leads to slow removal of waste products. Light activity and stretching continue the pumping action of muscles on veins, helping the circulation remove wastes. Also, the pulse should come down gradually by walking and stretching. Some experts believe that static stretching after the workout is more important than stretching before a workout, because it can help reduce delayed soreness or muscle pain felt the day after exercise.

Teaching Tips

Model with the entire class. Organize students into groups. Each group will work together to create a short act that will demonstrate the three components of a workout. Each group can use the clock to demonstrate the time lapse in each phase of the workout. Make a personal clock with a paper plate, cardboard hands, and a brad. Have students set the time at the beginning of the workout and move the hands after each component. Have students figure the total time for working out.

Lesson 7

Stick to It

Goals

- To improve cardiovascular fitness
- To introduce the concept of pacing

Key Concepts

One characteristic of a workout is continuous exercise for 20 minutes. This can be done in a variety of ways. Many children and adults find running is an easy way to accomplish a workout because no equipment is needed and it is an economical way to obtain moderate to vigorous exercise.

Materials

1. Popsicle sticks
2. Cones (eight)

Warm-Up: 5 Minutes

Select stretching and warm-up activities.

Activity: Stick to It

- Establish a 200-yard running area or, as facilities provide, mark out a specific circular or square running course.

- Students run continuously for a specific time around the course. The time period will vary according to age and endurance levels.
- First graders can run for four minutes and second graders for five minutes. Encourage them to run with one or two friends.
- Every time they pass the starting point, hand them a Popsicle stick. Have them count how many sticks they received.
- Give three or four minutes of rest for drinks, and repeat the run for the same time period. The goal is to reach the previous stick total.

Cool-Down: 5 Minutes

Select stretching and cool-down activities.

Teaching Tips

Model the concept of pacing and not going too fast at the start. Instead of sticks, you can keep track of the students' progress on a clipboard. You can ask children to predict their own performance (number of times completing the course) before the run, after you have described the course and the time period. Avoid using the word "laps" and refer to the "course." A child with a disability can run or walk with a buddy. Children with mobility problems can walk a shorter distance.

Lesson 8

Station Creation

Goals

- To introduce a station approach to exercise
- To develop cardiovascular endurance

Key Concepts

Stations are an effective way of providing continuous activity and organizing a large group for exercise. Student motivation increases through a variety of exercise choices.

Materials

1. Station cards
2. Optional equipment—jump ropes, soccer balls, basketballs, hula hoops

Warm-Up: 5 Minutes

Select stretching and warm-up activities.

Activity: Station Creation

- Divide class into groups of four or five.
- Set up six activity stations.
- Use exercises in chapter 13 to establish station activities.
- Other activities can include equipment such as jump ropes, hula hoops, soccer balls, and basketballs. For example, hula hooping for time, students try to keep the hoop around their waist for as long as possible. Students can try to keep jumping rope for as long as possible in the time period. With soccer balls and basketballs, set up a series of cones in a circle. Students keep dribbling in and out of the cones around the circle.
- Demonstrate each activity. Allow one minute per station and rotate groups.

Cool-Down: 5 Minutes

Select stretching and cool-down activities.

Teaching Tips

Vary the method by which students move from one station to another. Options include jogging, hopping, jumping in and out of hoops, animal walks (bear, lame dog, seal, rabbit hop). Include a station for a drink of water.

WEEK 2

Lesson 9

Start Walkin'

Goals

- To introduce a walking workout schedule to children
- To establish a walking program for children and their parents, friends, and families

Key Concepts

Walking has considerable lifetime value and is therefore worth introducing to children and their families. Walking is an easy-to-organize activity for children that they can do with family members. Walking with a partner or friend increases motivation and emphasizes the need for a support system for regular exercise.

Materials

1. Chips, Popsicle sticks, or Post-Its
2. Handout 2.2. Week 2, Family Activity: Walking Is Super Healthy (WISH) (one per student)

Warm-Up: 5 Minutes

Select stretching and warm-up activities.

Activity: Start Walkin'

- Map out a mile for a class walk. If there is no track available mark out a mile before class. You can use a track or a specific walking course in your school. Students can participate in calculating a mile course.
- The objective for this class lesson is for everyone to walk one mile.
- If you walk on a track, use chips, Popsicle sticks, or Post-Its to help students keep track of their progress.
- Clearly explain that this activity is a walk, not a run.
- Invite parents to walk with you.
- Use the class walk to establish a walking program for families.
- Use handout 2.2, Walking Is Super Healthy (WISH), to complete the home program.

Cool-Down: 5 Minutes

Select stretching and cool-down activities. Introduce and explain handout 2.2 Walking Is Super Healthy (WISH).

Teaching Tips

Students who are unable to get their parents to participate can complete their walking activities at school during recess, breaks, and lunch hour.

Model and explain proper walking technique:

- Shoulders are back and relaxed.
- Eyes are straight ahead and chin up.
- Strike down on front foot with heel as you push off with big toe of back foot.
- Swing arms naturally and rhythmically at sides.

WEEK 2
Lesson 10
Skim and Trim

Goals

- To describe how fat feels or tastes in food
- To recognize low-fat dairy products and the difference between whole, 2 percent, and skim milk

Key Concepts

All people need some fat in their diet—especially young children. But too much fat can cause heart problems later in life. Many foods have low-fat choices, such as the dairy group. You can get the same nutritional value out of milk (calcium, for example) whether it is nonfat or whole milk. So, one way to reduce fat in our diet is to drink skim or low-fat milk or dairy products instead of whole milk. You can eat less fat and still enjoy the good taste of milk, yogurt, and cheese. Fat in food, whether plant or animal fat, has certain properties that make food taste creamy, oily, greasy, and flavorful. If we can learn to recognize the taste, feel, and smell of foods that have fat, we can reduce the amount of fat we eat.

Materials

1. Three pitchers marked A, B, and C
2. Handout 2.1 Skim and Trim Taste Test (one per group)
3. Three types of milk—whole, 2 percent, and skim
4. Three paper cups (per student) marked A, B, and C to sample the milk

Activity: Skim and Trim

- Before class, set up the activity by pouring three types of milk into containers marked A, B, and C.

- Begin the lesson by reviewing the concepts learned in lesson 5. Tell the students that most plant foods are low in fat and animal foods are not. Can they describe what the fat in these foods tastes like (creamy, flavorful)? How does fat feel in the mouth (greasy, oily)? Can they describe how fat smells?
- Organize the students into small groups and give them handout 2.1. Explain to the class that there are three types of milk that will be taste tested.
- Describe the inquiry process to the class. First, they are to observe each of the three milks and discuss three terms to describe the appearance of each milk. Write or draw these terms on the handout. Next, have each student sample the milk. Write, draw, or discuss three terms to describe the taste of the milk. Then, after all three have been sampled, predict which has the highest to the lowest amount of fat.
- After all groups have finished, discuss results with the class.
- Show the class two healthy plants of the same kind to be used in lesson 15. Place both in a warm, sunny place. For the next week, water one but not the other. Be sure to record the amount of water you give to the plant.

Teaching Tip

If any of the students are allergic to or dislike milk, assign them the job of recording the data.

Handout 2.1   Skim and Trim Taste Test

Sample	Appearance	Taste
A		
B		
C		

Handout 2.2   Week 2, Family Activity: Walking Is Super Healthy (WISH)

Names _____

Week	Walk 1	Walk 2	Walk 3	Weekly total
1				
2				
3				

Dear Parents:

Try to walk three times per week over the next three weeks. Establish a walking course for your family. Put this sheet in a visible place (e.g., refrigerator) and keep track of miles walked. Estimate number of miles completed with each walk and for each week.

Time: 30 minutes per walk

Please return by _____.

Week 3: Fitness Components

Students complete tests of physical fitness components that provide baseline measures. In nutrition, the lessons introduce the essential role of water in health of individuals.

Lesson 11

Kinetic Kids

Goals

- To assess physical fitness levels of students
- To improve muscular strength and endurance and flexibility

Key Concepts

Cardiovascular (heart and lung) endurance, low-back and posterior thigh flexibility, and abdominal (stomach) strength and endurance are basic components of physical fitness. Cardiovascular endurance can help reduce heart disease, and flexibility and strength in the lower back and stomach can reduce low-back pain.

Materials

1. Stopwatch
2. Sit-and-reach box or yardstick or measuring tape and masking tape
3. Mats
4. Handout 3.1 Kinetic Kids Score Sheet

Warm-Up: 5 Minutes

Select stretching and warm-up activities.

Activity: Kinetic Kids

Test children on the following items:

1. **Half-mile run or walk** (cardiovascular endurance test)

    The score is the time to run or walk the half mile. Instruct students to run or walk at the fastest pace possible. Divide into pairs and complete in two separate groups with partners serving as recorders of time.

2. **Sit and reach** (lower-back and thigh flexibility test)

    Use a sit-and-reach box (see figure 3.1a) or a yardstick or measuring tape. If using a yardstick or measuring tape, put a piece of masking tape on the floor. Students sit per-pendicular to it with legs extended, knees straight, heels five to seven inches apart and just touching the inside edge of the tape. Place a yardstick or measuring tape between legs with the 15-inch mark on the inside edge of the masking tape. A partner holds the student's knees straight. The student places both hands on top of each other with fingers matching, then reaches forward with both hands as far as possible to touch the stick. Record the score to the nearest half inch.

3. **Sit-ups** (abdominal muscular endurance test)

    Student lies on back with knees flexed and feet flat on floor (see figure 3.1b). Heels are between 12 and 18 inches from buttocks. The arms are crossed on the chest with the hands on opposite shoulders. A partner holds the feet to keep them in contact with the ground. The student curls to the sitting position. Students must maintain arm contact with chest. The chin remains tucked on the chest. The sit-up is completed when the elbows touch the thighs. To complete the movement the student returns to the down position until the midback makes contact with the surface of the mat. The score is the number of correctly completed sit-ups in one minute.

Cool-Down: 5 Minutes

Select stretching and cool-down activities.

Teaching Tips

Students can work in pairs and take turns testing each other and recording scores. Students will obviously compare scores and there is a need to emphasize that scores are a baseline measure and improvement is the goal. This lesson is more than one 30-minute period. If time is limited focus on completing the half-mile run or walk. Use the scores from the fitness tests to introduce measurements scales. Students can do simple addition and subtraction with the scores from the fitness tests.

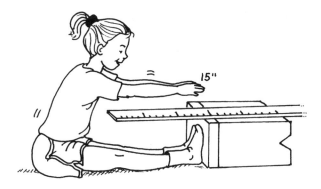

Fig. 3.1a   Sit and reach

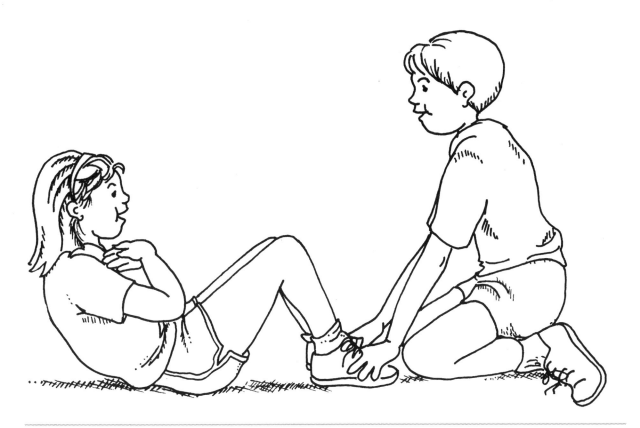

Fig. 3.1b   Sit-up

Handout 3.1   Kinetic Kids Score Sheet

Date _____

Name	Run or walk	Sit and reach	Sit-ups
_____	_____	_____	_____
_____	_____	_____	_____
_____	_____	_____	_____
_____	_____	_____	_____
_____	_____	_____	_____
_____	_____	_____	_____
_____	_____	_____	_____
_____	_____	_____	_____
_____	_____	_____	_____
_____	_____	_____	_____
_____	_____	_____	_____
_____	_____	_____	_____
_____	_____	_____	_____
_____	_____	_____	_____
_____	_____	_____	_____
_____	_____	_____	_____
_____	_____	_____	_____
_____	_____	_____	_____

Lesson 12

Workout Zoo

Goals

- To improve cardiovascular endurance
- To improve agility

Key Concepts

Students can learn the specific walking and movement characteristics of animals. Animals move at different rates for different purposes.

Materials

1. Four cones
2. Pieces of paper or cards with animal names or pictures
3. Small box for pieces of paper or cards

Warm-Up: 5 Minutes

Select stretching and warm-up activities.

Activity: Workout Zoo

- Demonstrate the walking and movement characteristics of the following animals—bear, lame dog, seal, crab, elephant, frog, and turtle (see figure 3.2).
- On pieces of paper, write the names of the animals.
- Set up four cones to make a 30 × 30 yard square.
- Spread children around outside of the square.
- One child picks a piece of paper and the class completes the animal movement around the square.
- Keep the pieces of paper in a box.

Cool-Down: 5 Minutes

Select stretching and cool-down activities.

Teaching Tips

Two smaller squares can be used to prevent overcrowding. At first children can practice each animal movement in turn until they have learned the specific movement. Once the students have practiced animal movements, have them vary the speeds with auditory cues (whistle, music). If children become overly tired, provide a rest or a walk around as a "human."

Lesson 13

Hoop Groups

Goals

- To improve cardiovascular endurance
- To improve coordination and motor skills
- To practice cooperative skills

Key Concepts

Emphasize cooperation within groups in this activity. The goal is to work together to move the hoop as a group while practicing motor skills. Cooperative games eliminate the fear of failure and the feeling of failure. They also reaffirm a child's confidence in himself or herself as an acceptable person.

Materials

1. Twelve hula hoops
2. Music and tape player

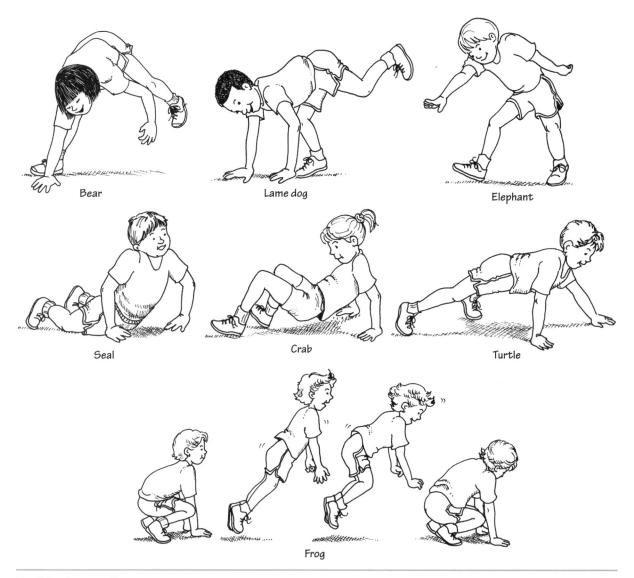

Fig. 3.2   Animal walks

Warm-Up: 5 Minutes

Select stretching and warm-up activities.

Activity: Hoop Groups

- Have each student get a partner and spread throughout the playing area (25 by 25 feet).
- Give each pair a hula hoop and have them get inside of it, holding the hoop at about waist level.
- When the music begins, the students skip around the gym.
- When the music stops, the pair must find another pair and get inside both hoops.

- The music begins again and now the foursome jog around the gym together.
- Change the locomotor skill to include jogging, galloping, skipping, and sliding.

Cool-Down: 5 Minutes

Select stretching and cool-down activities.

Teaching Tips

Emphasize group cooperation and safety. Devote more time to the first phase, two students in the hoop, and less time with four students in hoops.

This will allow more efficient practice of jogging, skipping, galloping, and sliding techniques. Children with mobility problems may not be able to skip, jog, or gallop. Allow them to move at their own speed, and the group in the hoop moves at that speed.

Lesson 14

Roll the Die

Goals

- To develop cardiovascular endurance
- To develop number recognition skills

Key Concepts

Cardiovascular endurance is combined with number recognition and practiced in an active format. The chance element in rolling the die to determine an exercise provides a motivational incentive to work out.

Materials

1. One die and a small box per three students
2. One chair per three students

Warm-Up: 5 Minutes

Select stretching and warm-up activities.

Activity: Roll the Die

- Divide class into groups of three with a chair 30 yards away from each group.
- On each chair place a box with a die in it.
- Describe and demonstrate the following six exercises (see chapter 13).

1. Coffee grinder
2. Crab legs
3. Cross-country skier
4. Mountain climbers
5. Jump twisters
6. Jack-in-the-box

- Students take turns running to the chair, and whatever number they roll determines the exercise for that group.
- The student yells out the number, and the waiting students in the group perform the designated exercise.
- The student returns to the group, and another student runs out to roll the die.

Cool-Down: 5 Minutes

Select stretching and cool-down activities.

Teaching Tips

Other exercises can be substituted. The children can use two die to practice simple addition and subtraction skills. Permit children with disabilities to perform alternative exercises. For example, a child in a wheelchair can perform arm raises instead of side leg raises.

Lesson 15

Water World

Goal

- To observe plants to introduce the role water plays in health

Key Concepts

Students will observe how important water is to the health of living things. Plants draw water up through the roots. Plants lose water through their leaves somewhat like humans lose water through their skin. Each of us should drink about six cups (48 ounces) of water a day to stay healthy.

Materials

1. Two plants, one that has been watered, one without water
2. Handout 3.2 Water World (one per student)
3. Bucket of water (one per group)
4. Paper cups (several per group)
5. Handout 3.3 Week 3, Family Activity: Something New

Activity: Water World

- Ask students to describe the differences between the physical appearance of the two plants by discussing, writing, or drawing their ideas on their handout.
- Discuss the differences. Ask the students what one plant was missing that the other one wasn't (water).
- Which plant would they describe as healthy? Which one is unhealthy?
- Then ask the students if they have ever felt healthy. What did they do? Have they ever felt water on their skin after exercising?
- What would happen to them if they didn't have any water to drink?
- When do they need to drink water? How often (when they are thirsty, throughout the day, after exercising)? Show the amount of water the plant needed per day.
- Have them "guestimate" and fill cups with the amount they need.
- Demonstrate the correct amount.
- Color the worksheet.

Handout 3.2   Water World

Plant   Draw each plant   Healthy (Y/N)

A

B

Color in the cups of water you need each day.

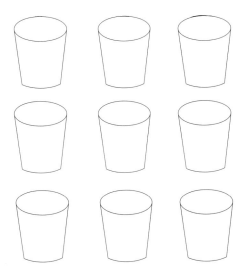

Handout 3.3   Week 3, Family Activity: Something New

For this week's home activity we would simply like you to try "Something New," or an activity that your family doesn't do very often. Call the family together and decide on one new activity or one you haven't done for a long time.

Examples

   Hiking on a local trail or beach
   Swimming at the local pool
   Bicycling
   Skating at a park or schoolyard
   Frisbee in the yard
   Bowling
   Running or jogging

   Many of these activities are free.

After completing the selected activity draw a picture in the space below of the family participating in the activity.

Time: 45 minutes

Return to school by _____.

CHAPTER 4

Week 4: Risk Factors

The lessons present the warning signs of a heart attack along with how to deal with an emergency. The activity lessons focus on individual risk factors.

Lesson 16

Help Is on the Way

Goals

- To teach warning signs of heart attacks
- To give practice dealing with emergencies

Key Concepts

Emergencies can happen at any time and place. Preparation for and knowledge of dealing with emergencies can save lives. Even young children can learn how to respond to emergencies.

Materials

A toy phone or real phone per group or figure 4.1

Activity: Help Is on the Way

- Teach the warning signs of a heart attack.
  1. Pressure or pain in center of the chest lasting more than a few minutes
  2. Pain spreading to shoulders, neck, or arms

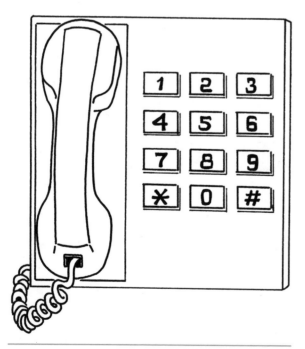

Fig. 4.1   Touch-tone phone

  3. Lightheadedness, fainting, sweating, nausea, or shortness of breath
- Explain what a heart attack is.
  A heart attack occurs when blood and oxygen do not get to the heart muscle and this hurts or damages the heart.
- The primary factors that may cause a heart attack are the following:
  1. Eating foods high in fat
  2. Smoking cigarettes
  3. Being inactive

  All these are controllable risk factors.

- Model the ways to deal with an emergency:
  1. How to assess the situation
  2. How to use the telephone
  3. What to say on the telephone
  4. How to provide comfort to victim
- Students can practice being an operator and caller. This would be a role-playing activity using a phone or figure 4.1. Use the following guidelines for callers:
  1. Give the phone number from which you are calling.
  2. Give the address or location and special directions to find the victim.
  3. Describe the victim's condition (for example, conscious, breathing, burned, bleeding, broken bones, etc.).
  4. Describe what happened, how many are injured, or what help is being given.
  5. Give your name.
  6. *Do not hang up!*

Let the emergency person end the conversation. They may have questions to ask or special information to give you about what you should do until help arrives.

Teaching Tips

Invite an individual who has experienced a heart attack to describe the symptoms and how he or she has modified his or her lifestyle. Visit a local police station for a demonstration of how local emergency systems operate.

Lesson 17
Plaque Attack

Goals

- To improve cardiovascular fitness
- To introduce the concept of unwanted plaque

Key Concepts

Plaque can stick to the walls of the arteries, blocking the blood's pathway. Plaque develops from fatty foods, attaches itself inside the blood vessels, and causes a blockage in the blood vessels of the body. The blockage may result in a heart attack or stroke.

Materials

1. About 25 to 30 foam balls (50 is ideal, however the game will work with fewer)
2. Twelve cones
3. Two boxes (optional)

Warm-Up: 5 Minutes

Select stretching and warm-up activities.

Activity: Plaque Attack

- In a gym or multipurpose room, divide the class in two groups.
- Mark a centerline dividing the room in half, with one team in each half.
- A team may not go over the centerline.
- Supply each team with an equal number of foam balls, which are in a big box or on the floor on their side of the centerline.

- On the teacher's signal, students begin throwing foam balls to the other side, *one at a time*, as fast as they can.
- Let them continue for a couple of minutes and then blow your whistle. All students must freeze.
- The side with the fewest foam balls (or plaque molecules) wins. Students divide up foam balls and start a new game.
- For a more active game, spread out the foam balls at the back of the playing area of each team.
- Students run from the centerline to the back of their playing area, then run to the centerline, then throw.
- Students can only get one ball at a time.
- When all balls are gone from the back of the playing area, the students may pick up a ball from anywhere on their side and run around a designated cone(s) away from playing area before throwing foam ball to the other side.

Cool-Down: 5 Minutes

Select stretching and cool-down activities.

Teaching Tips

You can use pieces of paper instead of foam balls. Make sure students do not throw balls at each other.

Lesson 18

The Healthy Highway

WEEK 4

Goals

- To improve cardiovascular endurance
- To reinforce the knowledge of controllable risk factors

Key Concepts

Two of the primary risk factors for cardiovascular disease are inactivity and eating fatty foods. Periods of inactivity are sometimes spent watching TV and eating high-fat foods.

Materials

1. Cones or tape to mark playing area
2. Foam balls for taggers
3. Pinnies for tagger identification

Warm-Up: 5 Minutes

Select stretching and warm-up activities.

Activity: The Healthy Highway

- Set up a playing area as shown in figure 4.2.
- Students must move from the safe areas through each risk factor area without being tagged.
- Their final destination is the land of health.
- Each inactive zone has one tagger.
- If students are tagged, they go back to the start but stay outside the cones, so not to interfere with runners.

Cool-Down: 5 Minutes

Select stretching and cool-down activities.

Teaching Tips

Play several small games of this activity. Provide each tagger with a foam ball. You can increase the number of taggers to two or three in each area.

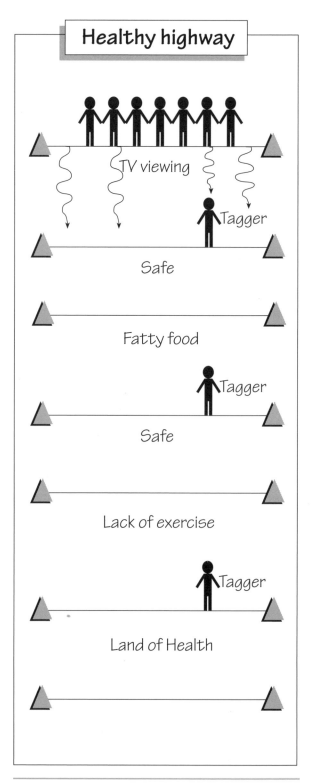

Fig. 4.2   The healthy highway

Lesson 19

Hospital Tag

Goal

- To improve cardiovascular endurance

Key Concepts

The goal for this lesson and others that aim to improve cardiovascular endurance is to keep children moving vigorously for 20 minutes.

Materials

1. Two foam balls for taggers
2. Cones to mark playing area

Warm-Up: 5 Minutes

Select stretching and warm-up activities.

Activity: Hospital Tag

- Designate one or two students to be the tagger(s). The other students spread out around the playing area.
- On a signal, the tag game begins.
- When a student gets tagged, he or she must hold that area with one hand. For instance, if a student were tagged on the back, he or she must hold that spot and not let go.
- The student continues to run, trying not to get tagged. If tagged a second time, student holds that spot but keeps moving.
- If tagged a third time, student freezes and shouts "9-1-1."
- Another student may help the injured player by doing 10 jumping jacks side by side. Students performing jumping jacks cannot be tagged.
- Taggers cannot stand by a pair waiting for them to finish.

Cool-Down: 5 Minutes

Select stretching and cool-down activities.

Teaching Tips

Adjust the number of jumping jacks to the ability of the students. Five may be enough for younger students. Use a foam ball for the taggers, who tag between shoulder and waist. You can substitute other exercises for jumping jacks.

Lesson 20

Growing Healthy

Goals

- To introduce students to alternatives to salt for seasoning foods
- To observe plant growth and the basic requirements to sustain plant life

Key Concepts

Salt provides flavor to foods, and our bodies all need some salt but not nearly as much as many people eat. You can give flavor to foods using herbs rather than salt.

Materials

1. Sliced vegetables (for dipping)
2. Vegetable dip without added salt
3. Several varieties of herb plants (not seed packets)
4. Potting soil
5. Pots or containers

6. Handout 4.1 Plant Calendar (one per group)
7. Handout 4.2 Week 4, Family Activity: Good Snackin' (one per student)

Activity: Growing Healthy

- Describe the objectives of the lesson.
- Prepare the vegetable dip before class (or use as a demonstration).
- Have students sample vegetables and dip. Explain that the recipe contains no added salt. Why is this important?
- Organize class into groups and give students an herb plant for them to plant. Students can select a location to place their plant.
- Each group will complete handout 4.1, Plant Calendar care schedule for four weeks.

Teaching Tips

You can often obtain plants at reduced cost (or free) from local nurseries.

Plants could be placed in an outdoor garden plot that students can design and care for. You could integrate this lesson into science curriculum concerning life cycles.

Basic Vegetable Dip

Ingredients
1 8-ounce fat-free or reduced calorie cream cheese
3 T. skim milk
1 T. lemon juice
1/4 tsp. garlic powder (not salt)

In a mixing bowl, combine the cream cheese (softened), milk, lemon juice, and garlic powder. Beat by hand or with an electric mixer until smooth. Choose one of the following variations and add to mixture:

a. 1 T. dried whole green peppercorns, crushed
b. 1 small can minced clams plus 1 T. minced parsley
c. 2 T. dill weed, 1 T. instant minced onion, and 1 T. parsley flakes

Handout 4.1   Plant Calendar

Each week one student from your group will be responsible for watering and caring for your plant. Complete the schedule below and place it next to your plant for quick reference.

	Student	Date	Amount of water
Week 1			
Week 2			
Week 3			
Week 4			

Handout 4.2   Week 4, Family Activity: *Good Snackin'*

When you feel a need to snack use the following list of alternatives to choose from. As a family, plan three snacks for the week that are heart-healthy choices. Circle your choices and indicate the day you chose to snack healthy.

Instead of this	Try this
Potato chips or cheese puffs	Popcorn (no fat added) or pretzels
Doughnut	High fiber muffins
Ice cream	Low-fat or nonfat yogurt
Soda	Fruit juice and sparkling mineral water
Beef burrito	Bean burrito
Chocolate chip cookies	Graham crackers
Chocolate cake	Angel food cake
Canned fruit in heavy syrup	Canned fruit in light juice
Mini pepperoni pizza	Mini cheese and veggie pizza

Time: 15 Minutes

Please return by _____.

Week 5: Aerobic Fitness

The lessons introduce the concept of aerobic exercise. Aerobic activities such as running are compared to nonaerobic activities such as running between bases in baseball.

WEEK 5

Lesson 21

The Fitness Race

Goal

- To differentiate between aerobic and nonaerobic exercise workouts

Key Concepts

For short activities such as quickly running up and down a small flight of stairs, muscles do not need oxygen. However, the body is only able to produce muscle energy without oxygen for brief periods. Short, intense exercise such as a 40-yard dash are nonaerobic (without oxygen) activities. Continuous activities over an extended time that require the body to use oxygen are aerobic.

Materials

1. Picture cards of different activities from magazines and sports cards (one per student)
2. Book, *The Tortoise and the Hare*
3. Venn circle or a piece of yarn

Activity: The Fitness Race

Read the book *The Tortoise and the Hare*. Introduce students to aerobic and nonaerobic activities. Discuss the difference between the concepts listed here.

Aerobic (running, bicycling): continuous, rhythmic, able to breathe.

Nonaerobic (baseball, 40-yard sprint): short, intense, out of breath quickly. Relate story to concepts (tortoise was aerobic and hare not aerobic, see figure 5.1). Demonstrate the aerobic activity of jump rope.

Demonstrate a nonaerobic activity, running to first base or running up a short flight of stairs.

Using picture cards create a single Venn diagram of aerobic and nonaerobic activities. Using the yarn, make a large circle on the floor. Pass out the cards. Ask students to describe different activities and whether they are aerobic or nonaerobic. Students put picture of aerobic activity in circle and nonaerobic activity outside the circle.

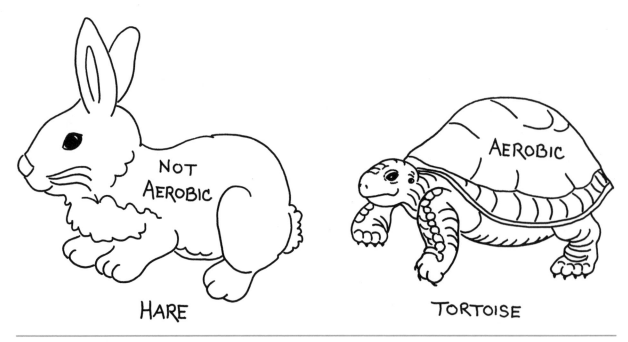

Fig. 5.1 Tortoise and the hare

Teaching Tips

Read the book ahead of time. Make up cards in advance. Older students who have already made sports cards (Family Activity from *Health-Related Fitness for Grades 3 and 4*) can supply cards. Students can role play action of tortoise and hare as story is read.

WEEK 5

Lesson 22

Tag Fest

Goals

- To improve cardiovascular endurance
- To reinforce aerobic and nonaerobic concepts
- To emphasize fair play

Key Concepts

Continuous and rhythmic exercise increases breathing and therefore the lungs take in more oxygen. This oxygen is then transported to the heart in the blood system and distributed to muscles to enable them to keep working. Tag games can be a combination of aerobic and nonaerobic exercise. Emphasize that students can play tag games in either an aerobic or a nonaerobic way. To play aerobically, have students moving at all times and not standing around.

Materials

1. Cones
2. Six Nerf balls
3. Whistle

Warm-Up: 5 Minutes

Select stretching and warm-up activities.

Activity: Tag Fest

- In Tag Fest, play a variety of tag games, changing formats about every five minutes.
- Establish a specific area for each tag game with cones.
- Give taggers a Nerf ball to tag other players with.

1. **Freeze tag**
   Designate three or four taggers. The objective is to tag everyone with a Nerf ball. Once a player is tagged, he or she stands still with feet apart and hands held above head. Free players can release the tagged players by crawling through their legs. A variation of this tag game is to have players dribble a soccer ball. To release tagged players, soccer balls or basketballs are dribbled through the legs of the frozen player.

2. **Back to back tag**
   Use an odd number of players. Start with players back to back except one player. On the command "jog," players jog in the playing area. On the command "back to back," all players find a new player to go back to back with. The remaining player keeps jogging.

3. **Elbow tag**
   Players pair up except one tagger, with elbows locked together and free hands on hips. The tagger tries to hook onto the outside elbow of a pair, while pairs try to avoid tagger. When the tagger hooks on the player on the other side becomes the tagger. You can use more than one tagger.

4. **Ten-second tag**
   Divide class in half with one group inside a playing area and the second group lined up along one line (see figure 5.2). On signal, two players from the line (the first two) run inside and have 10 seconds to tag a student. If successful, they trade places; if not, they get back in line.

Cool-Down: 5 Minutes

Select stretching and cool-down activities.

Teaching Tips

Emphasize tagging without pushing or shoving. Also, reinforce honesty and playing fair.

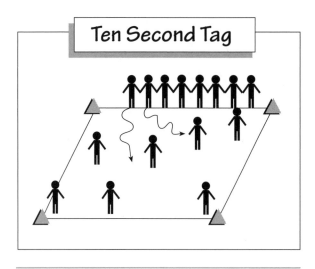

Fig. 5.2 Ten-second tag

WEEK 5

Lesson 23
Dice Day

Goals

- To improve cardiovascular fitness
- To practice mathematical skills
- To improve strength and endurance

Key Concepts

Rolling dice provides an effective motivational strategy and an opportunity to practice basic addition skills while exercising.

Materials

1. Two dice
2. One paper bag
3. Pieces of paper
4. Optional equipment—balls, jump ropes, hoops

Warm-Up: 5 Minutes

Select stretching and warm-up activities.

Activity: Dice Day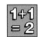

- Write specific activities or exercises on pieces of paper, fold, and put into a paper bag.

- Select activities or exercises that are suitable for the playing area.
- If limited space is available use exercises described in chapter 13.
- If a larger outdoor space is available, you can use more vigorous running activities.
- Have a student come up and pick a piece of paper from the bag. Teacher reads the slip aloud to the class.
- Then, have the student roll the dice. That's how many times the students must perform the task. For example, if "jumping jacks" was picked and a six was rolled, students complete six jumping jacks.
- When that task is completed, have a new student come up and pick out a new task, then roll the dice.

The following are examples: run around the perimeter of the playing area; push-ups; jumping jacks; touch your elbow to the opposite knee; clappers; mountain climbers; side leg raises; crab kicks; and jump rope; in groups of three, pass ball to each other while running a lap of the playing area; roll hoop around perimeter of gym. Do other exercises from chapter 13.

Cool-Down: 5 Minutes

Select stretching and cool-down activities.

Teaching Tips

Use the following developmental levels:

First graders—use one die and perform the number of exercises indicated on die.

Second graders—roll two dice and add the sum to indicate the number of repetitions.

Lesson 24
The Numbers Game

WEEK 5

Goals

- To improve cardiovascular endurance
- To practice ball skills

Key Concepts

One myth about exercise is that it can wear out your heart. An associated fallacy is that a person has a certain number of heartbeats in a life span. Exercise actually strengthens the heart. The heart muscle becomes thicker and stronger.

Materials

1. Ten playground balls
2. Ten cardboard boxes
3. Four cones

Warm-Up: 5 Minutes

Select stretching and warm-up activities.

Activity: The Numbers Game

- Set up an area 40 × 30 yards with four cones as shown in figure 5.3.
- Number students one to five (so five or six students have the same number).
- Students jog, walk, hop, skip, or run around the outside of the playing area.
- Call out a number, for example, four, and the number fours enter the playing area from either end. The remaining students keep moving.
- Students collect balls from the boxes placed at the ends of the playing area and basketball

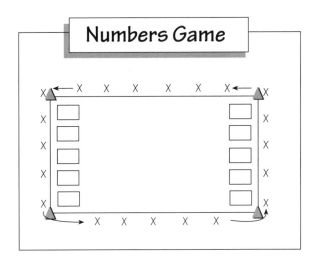

Fig. 5.3   *The numbers game*

dribble to the other end of the playing area. They place the balls in the boxes at the other end and rejoin the group on the outside.

Cool-Down: 5 Minutes

Select stretching and cool-down activities.

Teaching Tips

Change the type of movement with the ball (e.g., soccer dribble). Start with the group on the outside walking and increase to jogging. Place a number on each box so students can see that they deposit their ball in the box with the same number at the other end of the court.

Lesson 25

Rainbow Recipe

WEEK 5

Goals

- To introduce nutritional value to food color
- To encourage students to eat a greater variety of fruits and vegetables daily

Key Concepts

Fruits and vegetables are excellent sources of essential vitamins and minerals that we need daily to strengthen the body and provide energy. Many vitamins are pigments, such as B vitamins, and give color to foods like those found in the rainbow. By eating a variety of fruits and vegetables each day, or each color of the rainbow every day, we can be assured of getting enough vitamins and minerals. In this lesson, students will create a classroom bulletin board to demonstrate the spectrum of colors represented by fruits and vegetables.

Materials

1. Three-by-five cards
2. Crayons
3. Handout 5.1 Rainbow Recipe (one per student)
4. Variety of magazines containing food ads and recipes (or use the food picture cards from lesson 5 or students can draw and color their own)
5. Scissors
6. Rainbow-colored paper (sheets)
7. Tag board
8. Stapler, glue sticks, or push pins
9. Handout 5.2 Week 5, Family Activity: Playground Workout (one per student)

Activity: Rainbow Recipe

- Construct a bulletin board rainbow before class entitled "The Five a Day Plan." Include the rainbow colors shown in figure 5.4
- The product will be a bulletin board that will be approximately four feet by five feet. You'll

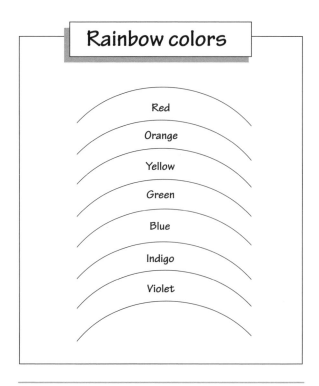

Rainbow colors

Red

Orange

Yellow

Green

Blue

Indigo

Violet

Fig. 5.4   *Rainbow colors*

need colored paper the colors of the rainbow. Cut the rainbow colors in an arc shape. You may need to piece it together if your colored paper isn't large enough. Glue or staple together the rainbow so it is one big piece. Overlapping each curved piece will be good enough, then glue. Staple 10 to 12 pockets on each curved color for the students to insert three-by-five cards into.

- Begin by describing the lesson objectives and content to the students by writing them on the board. For example, "Today we will learn . . ."
- Give the students handout 5.1 entitled "Rainbow Recipe" to explain the concepts. Guide the students to color the rainbow on the handout appropriately (red, orange, yellow, green, blue, indigo, and violet).
- Check the students' understanding by asking them to review the concepts orally.

- Lead the students through a discussion of which fruits and vegetables they have eaten that have different colors. For example, an apple is red; a squash is yellow, orange, or green; and an eggplant or purple cabbage is purple. Ask them to think of other fruits and vegetables that have the colors of the rainbow and write them on the handout. Other examples for red would include raspberries, red grapes, or red cabbage; blueberries or blue grapes for blue, and so forth.
- Assign each student to a group. Give each group several three-by-five cards, magazines with pictures of foods, and food picture cards. Instruct them to locate as many different foods that have the colors of the rainbow as they can. On a three-by-five card, cut and paste or draw the food, and across the top of the card, draw a line the color of the food. See the example in figure 5.5.
- Instruct the students to place the completed cards in the appropriate place on the bulletin board by color.
- Review the foods that each group found with the class.
- Discuss Handout 5.2 Family Activity: Playground Workout.

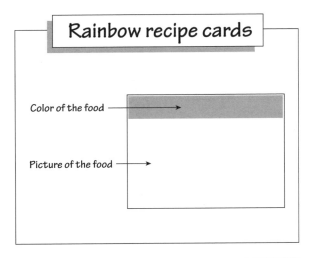

Fig. 5.5   Rainbow recipe cards

Teaching Tips

Make a transparency of handout 5.1 to make the rainbow for the bulletin board. The three-by-five cards will be used to plan a meal in lesson 30. Two books that you can use to integrate language arts are *Cloudy With a Chance of Meatballs* by Ron and Jan Barrett and *June 29th, 1999* by David Wiesner.

Handout 5.1   Rainbow Recipe

Color the rainbow.

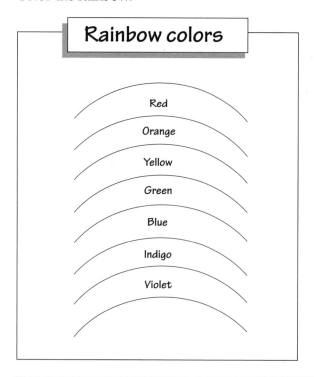

Rainbow colors

Red

Orange

Yellow

Green

Blue

Indigo

Violet

Fig. 5.4   Rainbow colors

Draw fruits and vegetables in colors of the rainbow.

Red   _____

Orange   _____

Yellow   _____

Green   _____

Blue   _____

Indigo   _____

Violet   _____

Handout 5.2   Week 5, Family Activity: Playground Workout

Often when children go to a playground, parents sit and watch. Tell your children to take their parents to the playground for a workout. Children and parents can work out together. Children and parents can complete the following fun activities:

Push-ups or hanging from the bars

Sit-ups on park bench

Jumping jacks in the sand

Step-ups onto a bench or piece of equipment

Knee lifts on parallel bars

Seesaw push down

Jogging or walking around the outside of the playground

Traveling on bar structures

Ask students to identify playgrounds in their neighborhoods and to describe play equipment. Set up a station workout, draw a diagram of the rotation sequence, and complete three circuits on next visit with parents.

Time: 30 minutes

Please return by _____ .

Week 6: More Aerobic Fitness

Students learn to take a pulse rate and have opportunities to practice this skill in activity lessons. The nutrition lesson presents fruits and vegetables as important sources of carbohydrates and nutrients.

WEEK 6

Lesson 26

Pump It Up

Goals

- To help children learn to find a pulse
- To demonstrate what happens to your heart when you exercise
- To demonstrate body responses to exercise

Key Concepts

The heartbeat is the sound of the valves in the heart closing as blood is pumped through the heart. The pulse is caused by the expansion and contraction of the arteries as the blood is pumped through them. Your heart beats faster when you are working and playing and slower when you are relaxing.

Materials

1. Four cones
2. Stethoscope (optional) or cardboard tube
3. Figure 6.1 How to Take a Pulse
4. Figure 6.2 (one per student)

Warm-Up: 5 Minutes

Select stretching and warm-up activities.

Activity: Pump It Up

Explain the following concepts to students: The heart is a pump. The heart is a muscle that never rests. The heart is in the chest and is about the size of a fist. The heart pumps blood to all parts of the body. What muscle works without you thinking about it? Demonstrate how to take a pulse using figure 6.1.

Mark out a square (30 × 30 yards) with four cones. Students pair up and play Ready, draw! (see chapter 11). After three to four minutes of activity

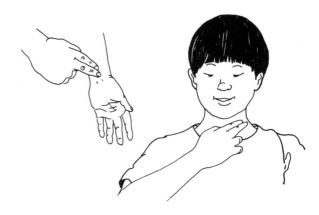

Fig. 6.1   How to take a pulse

ask children to locate a pulse as shown in figure 6.1. Children practice feeling for a pulse. Simulate the resting heartbeat by opening and closing the fist. Use the neck (carotid artery) and the wrist as locations. Children can take turns listening through a stethoscope to distinguish the type of beat they should be feeling. Play Ready, draw! a second time, then look at other reactions to exercise.

Explain the other physical reactions to exercise:

Perspiration—body's air-conditioning system

Heat and facial color—pump is working harder

Respiration—increase in breathing

Using figure 6.2 draw a picture of an activity that shows when the heart is pumping slowly and an activity (e.g., running) that shows a heart pumping rapidly.

Teaching Tips

Stethoscopes are often available from the American Heart Association. The room needs to be quiet to hear heartbeats.

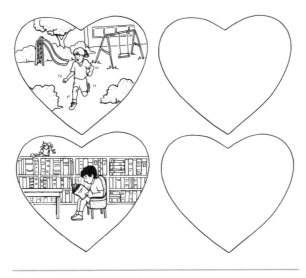

Fig. 6.2   A fast pump and a slow pump

Lesson 27

Hoopsters

Goals

- To improve cardiovascular endurance
- To develop cooperative skills

Key Concepts

Each pulse beat stands for one beat of the heart. Pulse rates rise during exercise and if you are excited, scared, or sick. Pulse rates are slow during resting, sitting, or sleeping. A boy's pulse rate is lower than a girl's pulse rate in most cases. A girl's heart is generally a little smaller.

Materials

1. One hoop for each student
2. Music and tape player

Warm-Up: 5 Minutes

Select stretching and warm-up activities.

Activity: Hoopsters

Variation 1—Island hoopers

- This game is like musical chairs, except hoops are eliminated, not players.

- The game starts with enough hoops scattered on the floor for all players, except one (or with large group, one hoop per pair).
- Players move around the playing area using a designated locomotion pattern, such as jog, skip, or hop.
- When the music stops, players must find a hoop (island) and freeze.
- Some hoops will have to be shared by more than one player as more hoops are removed. The object is to share space cooperatively until there are only three hoops left, and all players must work at getting some part of everyone's body in the remaining hoops.
- The focus should be on sharing and cooperating so everyone can find a hoop.
- Allow time for students to take a pulse rate.

Variation 2—Circle of hoops

- This variation involves using a circle of hoops (see figure 6.3).
- Divide your class into groups of five or six.
- Assign each group to a circle of hoops to begin the game.
- Each circle has enough hoops for everyone, minus one. Example: Four groups of six players per circle would need five hula hoops per circle.

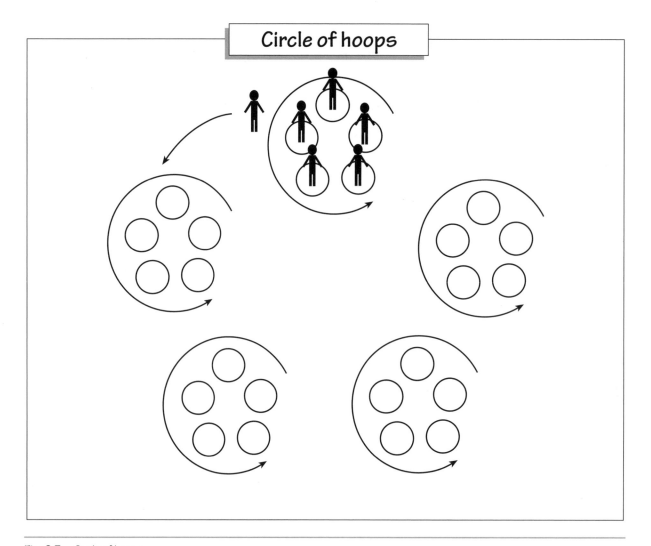

Fig. 6.3 Circle of hoops

- When the music begins, players move around the outside of their circles of hoops. When the music stops, all players must find a hoop.
- The player that does not find a hoop rotates to another circle of hoops (determine rotation before game starts).
- This variation keeps everyone moving and included in the game.

Cool-Down: 5 Minutes

Select stretching and cool-down activities.

Teaching Tips

Change movement patterns often. In Island Hoopers, you can remove more hoops, even down to one hoop if students remain in control. Compare the pulse rates of boys and girls.

WEEK 6

Lesson 28

Aero Hoop

Goals

- To improve cardiovascular endurance
- To develop cooperative skills

Key Concepts

Age will affect pulse rates. Newborn children have a pulse rate of about 130 to 140 beats every minute. First and second graders will average 80 to 90 beats per minute. The pulse rate lowers in the teenage years and stays the same throughout adulthood.

Materials

1. Four balls
2. Four hoops
3. Place markers (polyspots)

Warm-Up: 5 Minutes

Select stretching and warm-up activities.

Activity: Aero Hoop

- Divide class into four equal teams around the outside of a square as shown in figure 6.4
- Assign a hoop and a ball to each team.
- Give each student a number.
- Call out a number, for example, fives. Each number five runs to their team's hoop, picks up the ball, returns to their place, and runs around all the groups.
- Number five returns to own group and hands ball to number one in their group, who passes the ball to number two and down the line to the next player and finally to the last player, who returns the ball to the hoop.

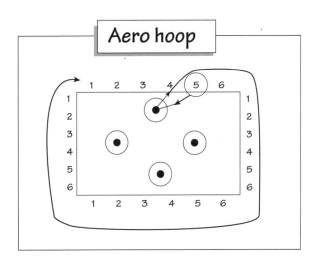

Fig. 6.4   Aero hoop

- While number five is running, the remaining players in each team complete an exercise (e.g., side leg raises, skiers, heel touches, stride jumps) specified by the teacher. The number of repetitions is the same as the number called out to run.
- Allow time for students to take a pulse rate.

Cool-Down: 5 Minutes

Select stretching and cool-down activities.

Teaching Tips

Use polyspots as place markers for students. Use exercises from chapter 13. As a variation, each student can have their own jump rope and jump while players are running. This activity can be a race, but emphasize performing exercises correctly. You can call out two or three numbers at a time and students can run together. If this is done, more balls are needed.

WEEK 6

Lesson 29

Hoop Aerobics

Goal

- To improve cardiovascular endurance

Key Concepts

The pulse rate tells you how fast your heart is pumping. Exercise makes the pulse rate go up rapidly. Most of the change takes place during the first two minutes. After that the pulse rate goes up more slowly and levels off.

Materials

1. One hoop per student
2. Tape player and music with a strong beat (optional)

Warm-Up: 5 Minutes

Select stretching and warm-up activities.

Activity: Hoop Aerobics

Students complete a series of hoop movements.

- Hold hoop vertically in front of the body and raise the hoop above head. Bend to the right and bend to the left. Repeat 10 times.
- Place hoop on the floor and step inside and jog.
- Hop in and out of the hoop. Change hopping foot.
- Jump in and out using two-footed jump. Jump three times inside, three times to right and left.
- Jump up and down three times, each time jumping a little higher.

- Jump forward out of hoop, back into hoop, backward out of hoop and forward into hoop.
- Place hoop on ground, run forward to hoop, and jump and land in hoop on two feet.
- Hoop jumping—use the hoop like a jump rope and try to jump five times.
- Hop all the way around the outside of the hoop, change feet, and hop around the other way.
- Hula hoop with hoop around your waist. See how long you can keep the hoop going.
- Toss hoop into air and catch. Start with a low toss. Repeat five times.
- Use the hoop as a steering wheel and jog around gym.
- Roll the hoop forward in an upright fashion. Run after hoop and repeat, keeping the hoop moving forward.
- Place all the hoops on floor and class jogs around playing area. Students can jump into hoop and balance on one foot for a few seconds, then return to jogging.
- Allow time for students to take a pulse rate.

Cool-Down: 5 Minutes

Select stretching and cool-down activities.

Teaching Tips

Demonstrate all movements and let students try each of the moves. Practice four or five in succession to make a sequence of hoop moves. Try performing moves to music. Students can select their own sequence of hoop moves. Each group can demonstrate their moves.

Lesson 30

Pick Pockets

Goals

- To plan a heart-healthy menu using the rainbow plan
- To reinforce the importance of eating a variety of fruits and vegetables each day

Key Concepts

Each group of students will plan a menu that contains a wide variety of fruits and vegetables. Challenge the students to create a meal with the greatest number of colors.

Materials

1. Cards from lesson 25
2. Handout 5.1 Rainbow Recipe from lesson 25
3. Crayons
4. Handout 6.1 Week 6, Family Activity: Home Run Cookies (one per student)

Activity: Pick Pockets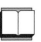

- Review the concept from lesson 25 that fruits and vegetables contain vitamins that color the food.
- Describe the objectives and content of the lesson by saying, "Today we will . . ." Establish the procedures for the lesson with the class.
- Demonstrate how to design or create a meal with a variety of fruits and vegetables using the bulletin board cards the students made in lesson 25. For example, a fruit salad could contain a variety of fruits. Add two or more vegetables to create a colorful meal.
- Place the students in groups to plan a dinner menu using the bulletin board cards.
- When they are finished creating their rainbow meal, ask each group to orally present their meals.
- Challenge the groups to design four more meals. Choose one to illustrate and color.
- Discuss and send home copies of handout 6.1, Home Run Cookies.

Handout 6.1   Week 6, Family Activity: Home Run Cookies

Try making these cookies for a heart-healthy family snack. By adding high-fiber ingredients and reducing animal fats, we can eat our cookies and be heart healthy too!

Ingredients

3/4 cup vegetable shortening
1/2 cup brown sugar
1/2 cup granulated sugar
2 egg whites
1/4 cup of water
1 tsp. vanilla
1/2 cup whole wheat flour
1/2 cup white flour
1/2 tsp. baking soda
1 cup raisins
3 cups rolled oats, quick cooking or regular

Directions

1. Preheat oven to 350 degrees.
2. Beat together the shortening, sugars, egg whites, water, and vanilla until creamy.
3. Combine flours and baking soda. Add to the creamed mixture.
4. Add raisins and rolled oats. Mix well.
5. Drop by rounded teaspoonfuls onto greased cookie sheets.
6. Bake 12 to 15 minutes.
7. Enjoy! (Makes approximately five dozen cookies.) Keep the recipe for future healthy snacking.
8. With your family, write your reaction to these nutritious treats. Return your responses to the teacher.

Time: 30 minutes

Please return by _____.

Week 7: Flexibility Fitness

Lessons 32, 33, and 34 include a special segment called Flex Focus. It emphasizes specific body parts in the warm-up for flexibility training. The purpose of this segment is to teach stretching exercises that improve flexibility for specific joints in the body.

Lesson 31

The Bends

Goals

- To introduce the concept that movements depend on flexible body joints
- To introduce the concept of ball-and-socket and hinge body joints
- To demonstrate the importance of body joints in everyday life

Key Concepts

Children learn to distinguish between ball and socket joints and hinge joints, recognizing that the type of joint determines what movement is possible. Other types of joints include gliding (forearm) and pivot (neck). Where the bones meet, they are cushioned by cartilage that prevents bones from crushing or grinding on each other.

Materials

1. Door hinge or a box lid (attached to box). Tape lid to one side of the box to simulate hinge action.
2. Joy stick from a video game, TV antenna, chair glide, or shower head
3. Foam or playground balls (one per pair of students)
4. Handout 7.1 Body Outline
5. Tape and four brads per student

Activity: The Bends

- Show students the two types of joints using the hinge and joystick. Help students identify the specific type of joints in the body.

  Hinge—elbow, wrist, finger, knee, toe, and ankle.
  Ball and socket—shoulder and hip

- Ask students which parts of arms and legs can move. Point out parts of body that have limited movement (back). Demonstrate that ball and socket joints (shoulder and hip) provide great flexibility compared to hinge joints (wrist and knee). Show how throwing a ball requires great flexibility (with a ball and socket joint) at the shoulder, enabling the throwing action to be completed.

- Organize students into pairs. Students can try to throw a ball but not rotate the arm at the shoulder. Point out the limited movement and range if the shoulder were fused and acted only as a hinge.

- Students can complete the stretches from routine 1 (p. 85) to demonstrate the amount of movement at the shoulder. Discuss how the arm can move. Also, point out how the shoulder needs to be very mobile to catch a ball. The hip is another example of a ball and socket joint.

- To illustrate the importance of a hinge joint movement, ask the students to demonstrate what their arm would be like if there was no joint at the elbow. Ask them to pick up and try and eat a food item without bending the elbow joint. Pose the following questions: How would mealtime be different? How would it affect food choices? Would you be able to eat soup?

- Children can cut out the various body parts (handout 7.1) and reattach using tape for hinge joints (elbow, wrist, knee, and ankle) and brads for ball and socket joints (shoulder and hip).

Teaching Tips

A skeleton (even a cardboard skeleton) is a useful teaching tool. To reinforce counting skills ask children to estimate the number of major joints of the arms and legs.

Handout 7.1   Body Outline

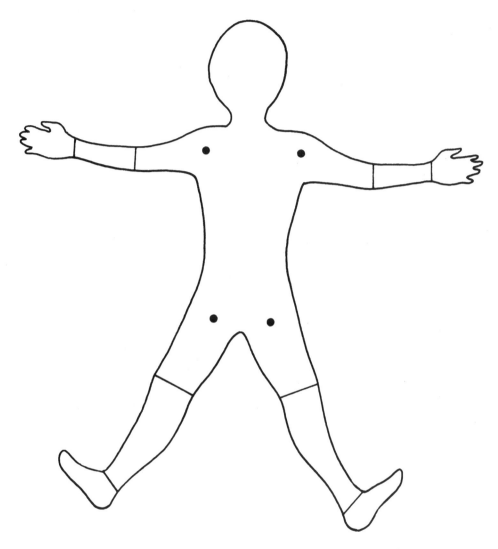

- Ball and socket joint
| Hinge joint

WEEK 7

Lesson 32

Paper Capers

Goals

- To improve coordination
- To improve low-back flexibility
- To develop cardiovascular endurance

Key Concepts

Few people make it through life without having lower-back pain. In most cases lower-back pain is caused by physical inactivity, poor posture, and lifting excessive weights. Lack of physical activity is the most common reason for back pain. Specific stretching exercises can greatly reduce the incidence and frequency of lower-back pain.

Materials

1. One piece of paper (red, white, or blue) per student
2. Tape player
3. Music

Warm-Up: 5 Minutes

Select stretching and warm-up activities. Give special emphasis to the chest and low back (see figure 7.2). Lessons 32, 33, and 34 include a segment called Flex Focus. Different body joints and parts are selected and specific stretching exercises are introduced for that joint or part of the body.

Flex Focus: Chest (see fig. 7.2)

1. *Chest stretcher*
   In a prone (lying on stomach) position, lift upper body off the ground so the arms are straight.

2. *Swimmer*
   Tilt the trunk slightly forward. Imitate a free-style swim stroke. Complete 10 to 12 strokes with each arm.

Flex Focus: Lower Back (see fig. 7.2)

1. *Sit and reach*
   Sit with knees slightly bent and feet pointed upward. Reach toward toes. Bend forward from the hips. Try to pull the chin toward the knees. Hold for 10 to 20 seconds. Repeat two or three times.

2. *Back stretcher*
   Pull the right leg toward the chest by holding onto the thigh. Keep the left leg slightly bent. Hold for 20 to 30 seconds. Switch legs. Repeat two or three times.

3. *Pill bug*
   Pull both legs to the chest by holding onto the hamstrings. Curl the head up toward the knees. Hold for 5 to 15 seconds. Repeat two or three times.

Activity: Paper Capers

1. Paper patterns
   - Divide class into three groups, one with blue pieces of paper, one with white pieces of paper, and one with red pieces of paper.
   - Organize in a scatter formation.
   - Children place paper on floor and jog around gym to music. When the music stops, each student finds a piece of paper.
   - Students perform a designated exercise with the paper, for example, an inchworm with hands on paper (walk up with feet to meet hands), coffee grinder (one hand on paper, body moves clockwise), modified push-ups over paper, jumping over paper, bridge up over paper, or reverse push-up over paper. Vary the movement to include jogging, skipping, galloping, hopping, and running backward.
   - Use the color-coded paper to determine exercise and movement. For example, students with blue paper perform a modified push-up, then skip; students with white paper perform a coffee grinder, then gallop; and students with red paper would perform a bridge up and jog.

2. Paper chase
   - Students scrunch up a piece of paper and throw and catch the paper as they move around the gym.

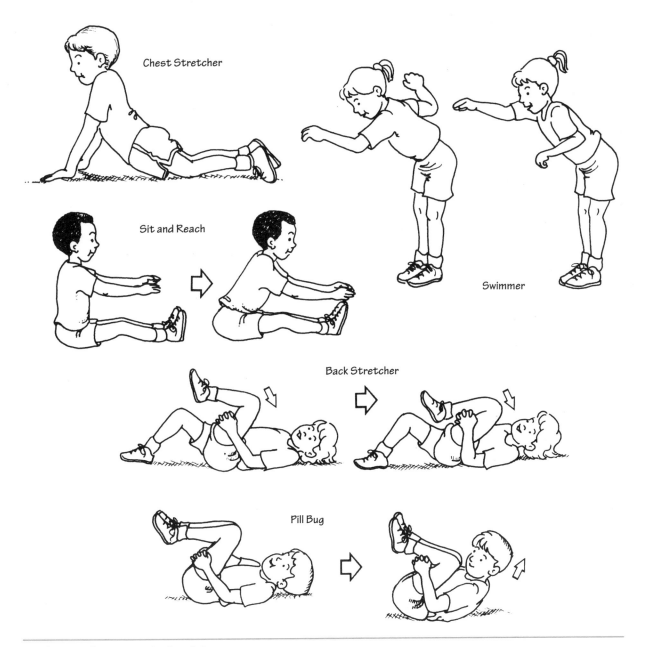

Fig. 7.2   Flex focus: Lower back and chest

- Use this movement concept to practice coordination activities. Throw and catch with one hand, throw and catch with right and left hand, throw and catch behind back, place on head and move, balance on foot and move, play catch with a partner, dribble like a soccer ball.
- Use the different colors of paper to emphasize different movements.

Cool-Down: 5 Minutes

Select stretching and cool-down activities.

Teaching Tips

Have a few extra pieces of paper available. Use exercises from chapter 13 in paper patterns to provide variety.

WEEK 7

Lesson 33

Flexible Friends

Goals

- To improve cardiovascular fitness
- To improve catching and jump rope skills
- To improve flexibility of upper legs

Key Concepts

Range of motion around a joint is highly specific and varies from one joint to another. Ligaments, tendons, muscles, skin, tissue injury, body fat, body temperature, age, and gender all can influence range of motion about a joint. However, the most important factor in improving flexibility is physical activity.

Materials

1. Fifteen bean bags
2. Fifteen playground balls
3. Cones

Warm-Up: 5 Minutes

Select stretching and warm-up activities. Give special emphasis to the legs (see figure 7.3).

Flex Focus: Upper Legs (see fig. 7.3)

1. *Sitting stretcher*
   Sit with soles of feet together, legs flat on the floor. Place hands on knees and lean forearms against knees; resist while trying to raise knees. Hold five to seven seconds, then relax.

2. *Hip and thigh stretcher*
   Place right knee directly above right ankle and stretch left leg backward so the knee touches the floor. If necessary, place hands on floor for balance. Press pelvis forward and downward and hold. Repeat on other side.

Flex Focus: Lower Legs (see fig. 7.3)

1. *Calf stretch*
   Stand with right leg forward and left leg back. Keep left leg straight and bend right

leg. Lean forward, keeping heel of left foot on ground. Repeat for right leg.

2. *Shin stretcher*
   Kneel on both knees, turn to right, press down on right ankle with right hand and hold. Keep hips thrust forward to avoid hyperflexing knees. Do not sit on heels. Repeat on left side.

Activity: Flexible Friends

- Mark out a playing area 30 × 40 yards.
- Give half the students a piece of equipment (bean bag or ball).
- Students jog in playing area.
- On a signal, students find a partner who does not have a piece of equipment and complete specific tasks. Provide a 30-second limit for the task.
- Students continue jogging for a specified time, then must find a new partner. The activity takes place between these two new players.
- Change equipment to other half of class after a while. Alternate between activity and specific stretches with partner and equipment.

Bean bag activities

Throw back and forth, throw with right hand or left. Catch with one or two hands. Throw high or low. Standing back to back, pass bean bag over head and through legs. Sit on floor and throw and catch. Vary distance between players. Emphasize success and playing so partner can catch the bean bag.

Ball activities

Throw back and forth using two hands to catch. Bounce pass back and forth. Basketball style shooting back and forth. Chest pass back and forth. Dribble toward and give to partner. Toss in air and strike with open hand to partner.

Cool-Down: 5 Minutes

Select stretching and cool-down activities.

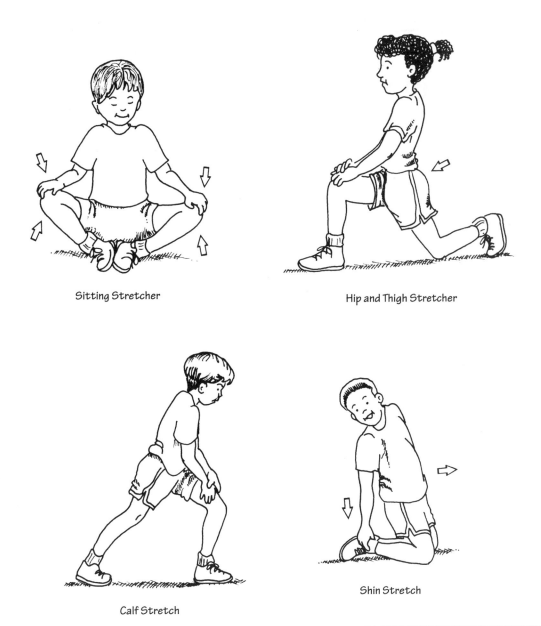

Sitting Stretcher

Hip and Thigh Stretcher

Calf Stretch

Shin Stretch

Fig. 7.3   Flex focus: Upper and lower legs

Teaching Tips

Demonstrate stretches before activity starts. Specify how far apart students should stand in bean bag and ball activities. Depending on skill level, use different pieces of equipment. Stress cooperation and proper use of equipment. You can use the equipment in this lesson for additional stretching activities.

Playground ball stretches

• Partners back to back, pass ball over head and through legs.

• Partners back to back, pass ball from side to side.

Bean bag stretches

• One partner lies on stomach and catches bean bag gently tossed by other partner. Hands are extended in front of head.

WEEK 7

Lesson 34

Jump to It

Goals

- To improve cardiovascular endurance through individual rope jumping
- To improve muscular endurance
- To improve coordination
- To improve neck flexibility

Key Concepts

Individual rope jumping emphasizes basic turning skills that serve as a foundation for jumping rope. Individual rope jumping is a valuable activity for physical fitness development because it can be completed at the discretion of the individual.

Materials

One jump rope for each student

Warm-Up: 5 Minutes

Select stretching and warm-up activities. Give special emphasis to the neck and shoulder (see figure 7.4).

Flex Focus: Neck (see fig. 7.4)

1. Neck stretch
Keeping shoulders back and spine straight, slowly roll the head to the left shoulder, straighten, then roll toward right shoulder, straighten. Repeat five times. Do not roll the head in a fast, circular manner or roll head backward.

Flex Focus: Shoulder (see fig. 7.4)

1. Shoulder shrug (helps to reduce muscle tension in neck and shoulders)
Shrug both shoulders up toward your ears. Hold and repeat. Shrug shoulders forward as far as possible. Hold and repeat. Shrug shoulders backward as far as possible. Hold and repeat. Shrug each shoulder opposite ways, up and down. Hold and repeat.

2. Reach for the stars
Hold both hands together and reach above the head.

3. Shoulder squeeze (stretches back of arms and shoulders)
Hold both hands behind your back (standing position). Straighten the arms. Lift the arms up and away from the back. Try not to lean forward (repeat two or three times).

Activity: Jump to It

Beginning skills

1. **Side swing**
Swing the rope held with both hands to one side of the body, then to the other side.

2. **Basic steps** (two and one foot)
Jumper jumps over rope with two feet as it passes under the feet. In the one foot step, shift the weight alternately from one foot to the other. Alternate using only the right foot, then only the left foot.

3. **Toes in and out**
Jump with toes pointed in and with toes pointed out. Alternate toes in and out or perform three in and three out.

4. **Backward jump**
Turn the rope counterclockwise and jump.

5. **Forward jump**
Turn the rope clockwise and jump.

6. **Double bounce or single bounce**
Jump with a double bounce after rope passes under feet or a single bounce after rope passes under feet.

More advanced skills

7. **Combinations**
Using the forward jump and backward jump, double bounce and single bounce, right foot, left foot, and both feet, put together a series of jump rope moves; for example, forward jump, single bounce, right foot only; back-

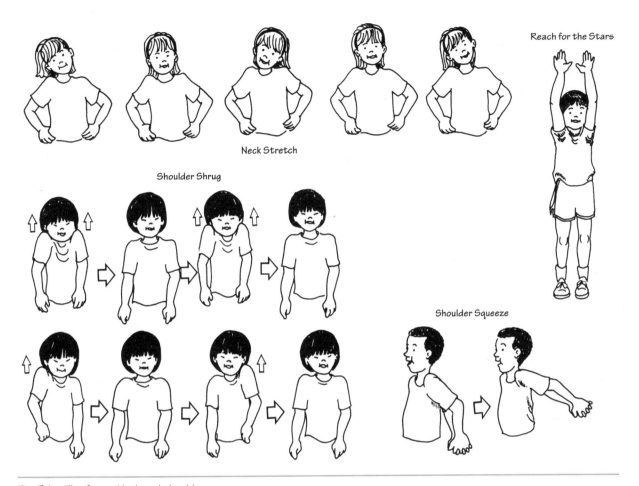

Reach for the Stars

Neck Stretch

Shoulder Shrug

Shoulder Squeeze

Fig. 7.4 Flex focus: Neck and shoulder

ward jump, double bounce, left foot only; forward jump, single bounce, both feet.

8. **Routines**
Set a goal for each student with 10 consecutive jumps for each routine. Students can put together a series of jumps using different formats.

Cool-Down: 5 Minutes

Select stretching and cool-down activities.

Teaching Tips

The rope should be long enough so the handles reach to the armpits. Hold the rope with the index finger and thumb on each side with the hands making a small circle when turning the rope. Em-

phasize that students do not need to jump high to clear the rope. Jumping rope for extended periods is demanding. Students can be partnered to allow for rest and recovery. Gradually increase jumping periods starting at 30-second intervals. Beginning jumpers may need to practice without a rope and to learn jumping and hand movements.

Jump rope stretches

- The jump rope can be used for additional stretching.
- Partners V-sit facing each other with feet touching. Rope is folded in half and partners gently lean forward and backward in opposition to each other.
- Partners stand shoulder to shoulder with feet and arms apart, holding rope in arms overhead. They move gently together from side to side.

Lesson 35

Time for Breakfast

Goals

- To reinforce the importance of eating breakfast daily
- To establish an appropriate eating pattern
- To practice time concepts and skills

Key Concepts

The body needs a constant supply of food to be healthy. Breakfast replenishes fuel sources after a long period without food. Breakfast provides the energy needed to work and play throughout the day.

Materials

1. Brads (one per student)
2. Paper plates (one per student)
3. Scissors
4. Markers
5. Construction paper
6. Handout 7.2 Time for Breakfast (one per student)
7. Large clock for teacher to demonstrate
8. Handout 7.3 Week 7, Family Activity: Vegetable Investigation (one per student)

Activity: Time for Breakfast

- Give each student the materials they need to make a clock with moveable hands. Use the paper plate as the clock face, construction paper to make the hands of the clock, and the brad to attach the hands to the clock.
- Ask the students to predict how many times per day their bodies need food. Students record their answers on handout 7.2 (or they can orally respond). Instruct the students to set their clocks to the time they ate breakfast that morning and record that time on the record sheets.
- Next, demonstrate and have the children move the hands to indicate what time the students ate their morning snack. How much time has elapsed between breakfast and the morning snack? Record this time and the difference on the record sheet.
- Throughout the day, use your clock to count the time that passes between meals and snacks. Be sure to keep track of the time between the last meal of the day and breakfast the following morning.
- Instruct the students to take the handout home to complete the activity.

Teaching Tips

First grade students should manipulate their clocks in hour increments.

Handout 7.2   Time for Breakfast

How many times per day do you need food? _____

Time   **How many hours between meals?**

I ate breakfast_____

I ate morning snack_____   _____

I ate lunch_____   _____

I ate afternoon snack_____   _____

I ate dinner_____   _____

I ate breakfast_____   _____

Handout 7.3   Week 7, Family Activity: Vegetable Investigation

The objective in this week's family activity is to try eating two new vegetables as part of your family's meals. Choose a vegetable that you have never eaten before. Find a recipe and prepare it with your family. After eating the vegetable, write a short description of the vegetable, including its name, color, how you prepared it, and what it tastes like. Under comments indicate whether you liked it or not.

Vegetable Investigation 1

Description

Comments

Vegetable Investigation 2

Description

Comments

Time: 30 minutes

Please return by _____.

Week 8: Strength Fitness

Lessons 37, 38, and 39 include a special segment called Muscle Moment. It emphasizes specific body parts in the warm-up for strength training. The purpose of this segment is to teach exercises that increase strength of specific areas of the body.

WEEK 8

Lesson 36
Mighty Muscle Measures

Goals

- To introduce the relative size and location of the major muscle groups
- To introduce and practice measuring skills

Key Concepts

Different muscle groups have different girths related to the function and location of muscles. For example, stomach and chest muscles are large to support and protect internal organs. Finger muscles are small to allow fine coordinated movements.

Materials

1. One piece of string (two yards) for each student
2. Scissors (one per pair of students)
3. Masking tape and markers to label strings
4. Body outlines (from lesson 1)

Activity: Mighty Muscle Measures

- Pair up students. Students take turns measuring their partner's major muscles using string.

- Students cut a length of string equal to the girth of the following major muscles.
    1. Upper arm (UA)
    2. Waist (W)
    3. Chest (C)
    4. Upper leg (UL)
    5. Lower leg (LL)
    6. Index finger (F)
- Label each piece of string (as they cut) with masking tape using the key just listed.
- Have students sort and arrange strings from shortest to longest.
- Select a volunteer to tape their strings to the chalkboard for discussion.
- Students tape or tie their strings in loops and attach them to the appropriate place on their body outlines.
- Discuss measurement results. Ask questions, "Why is the upper leg measure greater than the upper arm? Why do the waist and chest have greater girth than arms and legs?"

Teaching Tips

Helpers (parents or older students) can provide guidance. Emphasize the concept of the larger the string, the bigger or stronger the muscle. Pairing by gender may be appropriate.

WEEK 8

Lesson 37
Inflatable Muscles

Goals

- To reinforce names and locations of body parts containing major muscle groups

- To develop cardiovascular endurance
- To improve strength of chest, upper arm, and shoulder muscles

Key Concepts

The human body has more than 600 muscles. Muscles consist of reddish fibers that have great powers of contraction. The contraction and relaxation of muscles enables the body to move and perform coordinated skills such as running and jumping. The body's shape is defined by muscles.

Materials

1. One balloon per pair
2. Music (optional)
3. Tape player (optional)

Warm-Up: 5 Minutes

Select stretching warm-up activities. The muscle moment features a specific body part and provides exercises to strengthen that part. Give special emphasis to the chest, upper arms, and shoulders following the warm-up.

Muscle Moment: Arms and Shoulders

The triceps muscle is on the back of the upper arm. The push-up uses the triceps muscle to help lift you off the floor. The biceps muscle is on the front of the upper arm and allows you to curl your arm and bend your elbow. As you eat food, the biceps muscle allows you to move the fork to your mouth. The deltoid muscle helps lift objects and is used in throwing. Complete the following to strengthen these three muscles. See chapter 13 for exercise descriptions.

Crab legs

Support weight on hands and feet. Extend right leg forward. Extend left leg as right leg is brought back. Return to starting position.

Crab walker

Support weight on hands and feet. Move right hand and left foot forward simultaneously. Move left hand and right foot forward simultaneously.

Side standers

Student lies in prone position with chest touching floor, legs and feet together. Hands are directly under shoulders. Raise body in push-up fashion. At full arm extension, rotate body one-fourth turn to left, supporting weight on right hand and foot. Return to starting position. Rotate body to the right, supporting weight on the left hand and foot. Return to starting position.

Muscle Moment: Chest

The main chest muscles are the pectorals. The pectorals are shaped like a fan and help to cover and protect the upper ribs. The pectorals help you pull the arm across the front of the body. They are used in hugging. See chapter 13 for exercise descriptions.

Push-ups or modified push-ups

Lie on stomach with chest touching the floor and feet together. Hands are under the shoulders. Push and raise body by extending arms. Raise body in straight line from the knees, not allowing back to sway. Lower body until chin touches ground.

Activity: Inflatable Muscles I

- Divide class into pairs.
- Each pair keeps their balloon in the air by using body parts.
- Call out the body part, for example, shoulder. Students can only use the shoulder to keep the balloon in the air. Call out the names of different body parts.
- Ask students to move the balloon the length of the activity area.
- Group students in fours with two balloons moving simultaneously.

Activity: Inflatable Muscles II

- Organize students in groups of five with three on one side and two on the other.
- First student from group of three takes balloon across to the other side and passes balloon to the first student in the group of two, who then takes the balloon across to the other side.
- Each time the student transporting the balloon joins the back of the line.

Cool-Down: 5 Minutes

Select stretching and cool-down activities.

Teaching Tips

You will need extra balloons for those that pop. Use music to set the pace of the balloon moves. Use different colored balloons as an alternative grouping method. Save balloons for a science lesson on static electricity.

WEEK 8

Lesson 38

Return to the Hoop

Goals

- To improve cardiovascular endurance
- To practice basic ball skills
- To practice cooperative skills
- To improve abdominal and lower back strength.

Key Concepts

Strength is crucial for optimal performance in daily activities such as sitting, walking, running, lifting, carrying objects, and enjoying recreational activities. Strengthening the torso with exercises in this lesson will help reduce lower-back pain.

Materials

1. Four hoops
2. Twelve cones
3. Fifteen playground balls

Warm-Up: 5 Minutes

Select stretching and warm-up activities. Emphasize the abdominals and back following the warm-up.

Muscle Moment: Abdominals

The rectus abdominis or the abdominals support and protect body organs. The abdominals allow you to move your spine. Encourage children to start with five repetitions of each exercise. See chapter 13 for exercise descriptions.

Crunches

Student lies on floor legs together, knees bent, and hands across chest. Lift knees to elbows. Return to starting position.

Bridge backs

Student is on hands and knees in crawling position with feet shoulder-width apart. Tighten abdominal muscles and arch back as high as possible. Return to starting position. Emphasize importance of tightening abdominal muscles (students should feel it).

Reverse sit-ups (works lower portion of abdomen)

Lie on back with bent legs together and arms and hands extended over head. Bend at the waist bringing knees as close to the chest as possible.

Obliques (strengthens side of torso)

Lie on back with knees bent, feet on floor with hands held lightly behind head. Lift shoulder and upper torso off the floor twisting toward opposite knee. Do not pull head and neck with hands. Return to starting position and repeat on other side. Press spine to floor so hips do not roll.

Muscle Moment: Lower Back

The latissimus dorsi (shortened to lats) are triangle shaped and extend from under the shoulders to the lower back. Lift your right arm over your head and place your left hand under your right shoulder. Slowly pull your right elbow to your right hip and feel your lats muscle contract. The lats help you climb a rope. The trapezius is located on the upper back below the neck and lifts the shoulders up and down as in a shoulder shrug. See chapter 13 for exercise descriptions.

Curl-ups

In this exercise the lower back acts as a stabilizer. Lie on floor with hands on upper thighs, reach up until upper back comes off the ground.

Chest raises

In this activity, the lower back is a prime mover. Lie on stomach with arms at sides and raise chest and head from the ground.

Activity: Return to the Hoop

- In a large outdoor playing area, set up a square 40 × 40 yards with cones.
- Divide class into pairs with one student of each pair standing on the perimeter of the square. The other students stand inside the square about five yards away from their partners.

- Outside players run to hoop behind them (placed 30 to 40 yards away as shown in figure 8.1) to get a ball and return to face partner.
- Students complete a task (see following list) and the other partner returns ball to hoop. Partners then change positions.

Tasks

1. Roll ball
2. Pass back and forth (overhead, chest, underhand)
3. Bounce pass
4. Hike pass

Cool-Down: 5 Minutes

Select stretching and cool-down activities.

Teaching Tips

Prior practice and knowledge of ball skills is an advantage. Change partners throughout lesson.

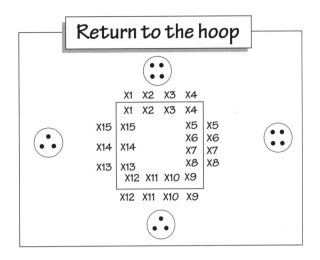

Fig. 8.1   Return to the hoop

Lesson 39

Rope Routes

Goals

- To improve cardiovascular endurance
- To improve jump rope skills
- To improve the strength of upper and lower leg muscles

Key Concepts

The American Heart Association sponsors Jump Rope for Heart. The American Heart Association lists physical inactivity or lack of exercise as a risk factor for heart disease along with cigarette smoke, high blood pressure, and high blood cholesterol levels.

Materials

Six to eight long jump ropes

Warm-Up: 5 Minutes

Select stretching and warm-up activities. Give special emphasis to the legs following the warm-up.

Muscle Moment: Upper Legs

The hamstrings are the muscles on the back of the top part of your leg. The hamstrings allow you to bend the knee. All running activities will use the hamstring muscles. The thigh muscles are one of the strongest muscle groups in the body. The quadriceps are on the front part of the upper leg. Quad means four and there are four long muscles that start near the hip and extend down to the knee. The quadriceps help you straighten your leg.

The following exercises use the quadriceps and hamstring muscle groups (in addition to others). Demonstrate the two exercises designed to strengthen the upper legs. See chapter 13 for exercise descriptions.

Stride jumps

Stand with feet together. Jump off ground so feet are spread about three feet apart. Then return to starting position. Similar to jumping jacks with no arm movements. Complete 15 repetitions.

Leg extensions

Kneel on the floor and place hands in front of body. Extend leg behind body and lift. Complete 10 repetitions with each leg.

Muscle Moment: Lower Leg

The calf muscle (gastrocnemius) lifts the foot up and down and is used to stand on the toes and balance. The following exercises use the lower leg.

Heel lifts

Lift heels off the ground, bend the knees slightly, and push off toes into an upright position. Knees should not go past a 90-degree angle. Complete 10 repetitions.

Ten jumps higher

Make a series of 10 jumps, each one higher than the previous one. Complete three repetitions.

Sprint starts

Start on all fours with the right knee forward. On command "set" students raise knees off the ground. On command "go" students sprint for 10 yards and slow down, completing a 20-yard run. Complete 3 repetitions.

Activity: Rope Routes

- Six pairs of rope turners (older students or parent volunteers) spread around area to create a circuit.
- Divide students into six groups and send them to a rope station.
- Rope turners turn ropes forward.
- Students jump through each rope three times, then jog to the next station.
- Vary movement between each station with skipping, galloping, side-to-side sliding, and hopping movements.

Cool-Down: 5 Minutes

Select stretching and cool-down activities.

Teaching Tips

This activity can be done outdoors, and the distance between stations can be increased. Include a water drink station.

WEEK 8

Lesson 40

Healthy Harvest

Goals

- To provide an alternate seasoning to salt
- To harvest and dry the herbs planted in lesson 20

Key Concepts

You can use herbs in place of salt to season foods. Dried herbs take more time when cooking to develop their full flavor. Fresh herbs are milder than dried and you need to use more herb to achieve the same flavor. For best flavor, harvest the herbs just before they blossom. Some herbs, such as basil, can be cut many times. Remove stems from small-leafed herbs like thyme. Harvest the herbs early in the day, if possible, picking only well-developed plants. Use scissors to cut the herb.

Materials

1. The herb plants students began growing in lesson 20
2. Plastic bags (one per group)

3. Towels
4. String (six inches per group)
5. Newspaper (one per group)
6. Old spice jars, baby food jars, or plastic Zip-loc bags (one per student)
7. Permanent markers (one per group)
8. Labels for jars or plastic bags (one per group)
9. Scissors
10. Handout 8.1 Week 8, Family Activity: Week-end Workout

Activity: Healthy Harvest

- Briefly discuss the key concepts with the class so they will understand before beginning the harvest.
- Demonstrate how to harvest the herbs (all the instructions follow).
- Instruct each group to spread out the newspaper; then give each group their herbs.
- Each group will divide their herbs in half. One half will be dried and the other half frozen. Use the following techniques:

To dry herbs

a. Use scissors to cut the herbs close to the dirt.

b. Make sure the herbs are clean by shaking off any dirt.
c. Tie the bunch of herbs with a string and mark them with each student's name.
d. Hang the herbs in a dark, dry area.
e. When the herbs are dried in a few days, crumble the leaves and place in small jars that are airtight and well sealed (old spice jars or baby food jars work well, or plastic Ziploc bags).
f. Mark each jar with the name of the herb and the student's name and date.
g. Keep the jars in a cool, dark place to use in lesson 45.

For fresh or frozen herbs

a. Use scissors to cut the herb close to the dirt.
b. Rinse them in cold water and wrap them in a paper towel.
c. Place these herbs wrapped in a towel, in a plastic bag and seal.
d. Make sure the plastic bag has the name of the herb, date, and student's name.
e. Freeze the fresh herbs.

Handout 8.1   Week 8, Family Activity: Weekend Workout

Take the family to the school track or a similar area. It's a perfect place to work out. Warm up by walking once around the track. Keep walking or break into an easy jog. Complete some stretches. If there are bleachers, stride up and down the bleachers to give the buttocks a workout. Then complete a series of exercises. Every 100 yards around the track, complete 10 repetitions of an exercise (such as mountain climbers, jumping jacks, cross-country skiers, stride jumps, or jump twisters). Your child can show you how to perform the exercises. Include four different exercises each lap. Walk or jog another lap and complete 15 repetitions of the same exercises. Cool down by walking a lap and doing some gentle stretching.

Time: 30 minutes

Please return by _____.

CHAPTER 9

Week 9: Healthy Lifestyle

Students receive encouragement to play active rather than inactive games. Planning and eating a heart-healthy meal is the culminating activity in nutrition.

WEEK 9

Lesson 41

Active Alternatives

Goals

- To help students recognize active alternatives to sedentary pursuits
- To distinguish between inactive and active games

Key Concepts

A great advantage the body has over other machines is that it is not worn out by use. Body parts and systems function better when they are active. When people have lain in bed for several weeks, bones lose minerals and become weak, the heart cannot pump as much blood, muscles weaken, and fitness declines. Therefore, physical activity can help maintain essential body functions.

Materials

1. Active Alternatives, figure 9.1
2. Foam balls (six)
3. Telephone

Warm-Up: 5 Minutes

Select stretching and warm-up activities.

Activity: Active Alternatives

Play an inactive game (e.g., Duck, Duck, Goose). Ask children to check for the physical signs of exercise (e.g., perspiration, heart rate—see lesson 26). Then play an active game (such as those in lesson 22) and ask children to observe their physical response to exercise. Hand out and discuss figure 9.1 with students and suggest alternative activities. Using pictures on figure 9.1 children can identify alternatives to the following: watching television, riding in a car, and riding an escalator. Children can draw active alternatives to these activities.

Discuss with students how they can make simple adjustments to achieve a more active lifestyle.

Cool-Down: 5 Minutes

Select stretching and cool-down activities.

Teaching Tips

Model a telephone conversation with students using a toy telephone or real phone (unplugged). The conversation concerns students getting together for an after school or weekend activity. Caller one invites the student over to watch TV or play a new video game. Caller two suggests an active alternative for the two to participate in or a reduced time watching TV or playing a video game. For example, I will watch TV for 30 minutes if we can ride bikes afterward. Teacher can make up key word cards for the students. Using props enhances the activity.

WEEK 9

Lesson 42

Parachute Power

Goals

- To improve cardiovascular fitness
- To improve arm, shoulder, and abdominal strength and endurance

Key Concepts

Parachutes provide a new and interesting means of accomplishing physical fitness goals with opportunities for improving strength, agility, coordi-

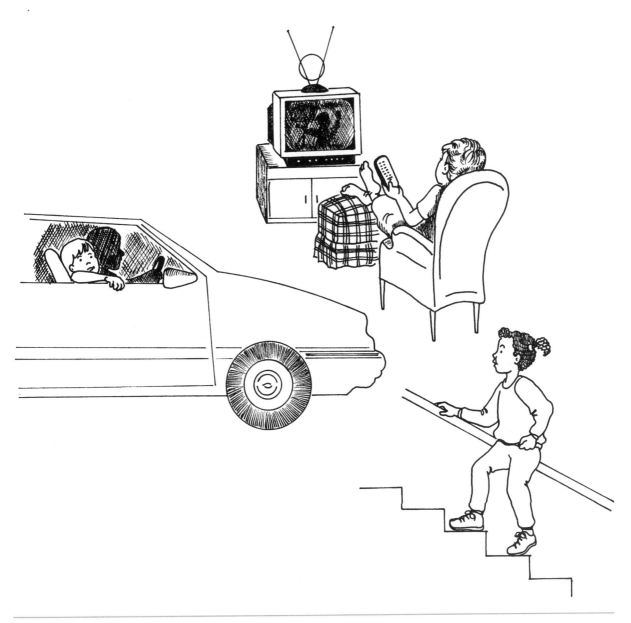

Fig. 9.1 Active alternatives

nation, and endurance. Focus strength development especially on the arms, hands, and shoulder girdle.

Materials

1. Nylon parachute with a diameter of 24 to 28 feet
2. Eight to ten foam balls
3. Plastic bags
4. String
5. Washers

Warm-Up: 5 Minutes

Select stretching and warm-up activities.

Activity: Parachute Power

Teach the grips for holding onto the chute—overhand (palms facing away), underhand (palms facing toward), or mixed (one hand underhand and the other overhand).

1. **Tidal waves**
   Students grip chute near outer edge with

hands, palms down, and shake vigorously. Keep elbows straight. Vary size of waves.

2. **Chute scoot**
   Grasp chute in right hand, move clockwise, and vary movements with skip, jog, run, hop. Switch hands and change direction.

3. **Popcorn**
   Place Nerf or rubber balls on chute. Shake well and try to bounce all balls off the chute.

4. **Keep on rollin'**
   Hold chute waist high and roll chute forward and then move backward, unrolling the chute.

5. **Parapull**
   All students pull chute at same time, leaning back and holding for 10 seconds.

6. **Strength stretcher**
   Students grasp chute behind back and face outward, while holding chute overhead. On signal, students hold and pull for 10 seconds.

7. **Cannonball**
   Place a ball in the center of the chute and lift

up slowly, then vigorously down on command to shoot ball toward ceiling.

8. **Sit-ups**
   Sit down with legs underneath the parachute, while grasping the chute with overhand grip. On signal, all students complete a sit-up. Repeat 15 times.

Cool-Down: 5 Minutes

Select stretching and cool-down activities.

Teaching Tips

Use cues, such as a whistle, to change directions. Chute Scoot should last 5 to 10 minutes. In Popcorn, designate a ball chaser. Students can make their own parachute by cutting open a plastic bag. Tie string to each corner and attach string to a washer.

WEEK 9

Lesson 43
Cardio Course

Goals

- To encourage children to cooperate and complete activities together
- To improve muscular strength and cardiovascular endurance

Key Concepts

There is mounting evidence that children who do not exercise are less likely to exercise as adults. Unless we teach children how to be physically active and to feel physically competent, they will not engage in active pursuits.

Materials

Twenty cones (different colors if available)

Warm-Up: 5 Minutes

Select stretching and warm-up activities.

Activity: Cardio Course

- Set up a circular course with cones as markers.
- A large indoor space is ideal, or use an outside grassy area.
- In pairs, students complete the designated activities as shown in figure 9.2.
- Describe course and demonstrate how to do the activities.
- Spread partners out on course and tell children not to pass the pair in front.

Activities

1. Partner skipping, holding hands
2. Follow the leader, who hops and skips
3. Cone slalom with hands on shoulders
4. Sideways shuffle with hands on hips
5. Three-legged walk (one person puts arm around shoulder of partner and hops)

Cool-Down: 5 Minutes

Select stretching and cool-down activities.

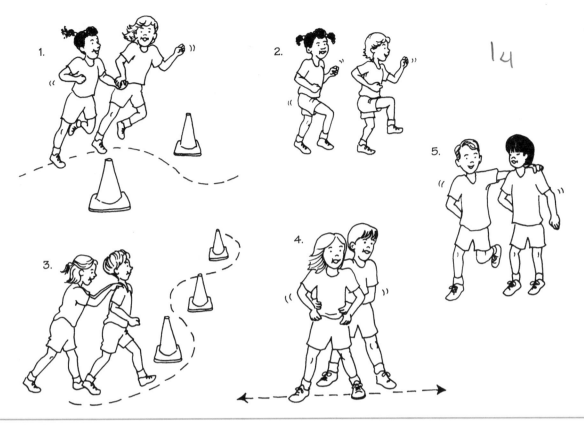

Fig. 9.2 *Cardio course*

Teaching Tips

Try to match pairs by gender and size. The objective is to move quickly and complete activities correctly. Encourage children to perform all activities as shown. After children are familiar with the activity, older students can change partners or reverse direction on the course.

Lesson 44

Circulatory Circuit

Goals

- To improve cardiovascular endurance
- To improve ball skills

Key Concepts

In spite of the public's knowledge of the positive effects of physical activity, only 22 percent of adults engage in leisure time activity at the levels recommended for health benefits. Possibly the low rate of participation is because the public perceives that they must engage in vigorous exercise. The scientific evidence shows that moderate physical activity can also provide substantial health benefits.

Materials

1. One ball per pair of students
2. Obstacles—cones, chairs, hoops

Warm-Up: 5 Minutes

Select stretching and warm-up activities.

Activity: Circulatory Circuit

- Set up an obstacle course with chairs, cones, and hoops as shown in figure 9.3.
- Pair up students with one ball per pair. Spread pairs around the outside of the course.
- Assign numbers 1 and 2 to each pair.
- Partner 1 moves through the course and around the obstacles. After one circuit, partner 1 exchanges the ball with partner 2, who then completes the course.

- The partner who is not on the circuit can complete designated exercises or walk/jog around the outside of the course.

Cool-Down: 5 Minutes

Select stretching and cool-down activities.

Teaching Tips

Spread out obstacles to allow space for dribblers, making sure there are no bottlenecks. Spread pairs out in course. Don't allow passing or overtaking unless the course is wide enough. If there is an odd number, make a threesome.

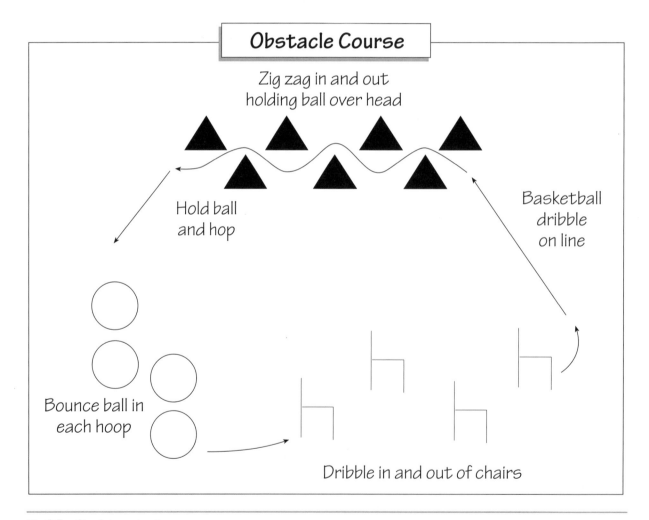

Fig. 9.3 *Circulatory circuit*

WEEK 9

Lesson 45

Final Feast

Goals

- To prepare and share a heart-healthy meal made with the herbs harvested in lesson 40
- To taste alternatives to salt as a seasoning

Key Concepts

As a culmination of the lessons on cardiovascular health, the students will prepare a meal and share with each group in a final feast.

Spaghetti Sauce

(serves 4)

1 medium onion, chopped (about 1/2 cup)
2 cloves garlic, minced
1 T. olive oil
1 can (1 pound) salt-free tomatoes
1 can (15 ounces) salt-free tomato sauce
1 T. parsley
1 tsp. oregano
1 tsp. basil

Sauté the onion and garlic in the olive oil until tender. Stir in the remaining ingredients. Heat to boiling, stirring occasionally. Reduce heat and simmer uncovered 45 minutes to 1 hour. Serve over spaghetti noodles.

Materials

1. Low-salt spaghetti sauce recipe made with the herbs grown and dried from lesson 40
2. Spaghetti noodles, bread, a fruit juice, and ingredients for making green or fruit salads
3. Paper plates and napkins, plastic eating utensils, and beverage cups (one per student)
4. Utensils for food preparation
5. Handout 9.1 Week 9, Family Activity: Family Triathlon (one per student)

Activity: Final Feast

- Divide the class into groups to prepare a fruit salad, a tossed green salad with colorful vegetables, spaghetti sauce, and spaghetti noodles.
- After all the groups have finished preparing their food, instruct them to put it on the buffet table. Before the class begins to eat, ask each group to identify how the food they prepared fits into a heart-healthy food category.
- Enjoy!

Teaching Tips

Arrange with parent volunteers to organize the materials. Schedule at least one parent volunteer per group to help the students prepare their meal. Instruct the students to designate a member of their group to collect the ingredients for their food to be prepared. While the students are preparing their recipe, set up a buffet table area in the classroom for the foods to be placed on when they've finished.

Handout 9.1   Week 9, Family Activity: Family Triathlon

A triathlon consists of running, swimming, and bicycling. Triathletes are recognized as being outstanding endurance athletes. Take the triathlon concept and have fun with your family. Choose three activities that your family enjoys, such as walking, bicycling, jogging, jumping rope, soccer, basketball, touch football, or others. Select the three sports or activities to do one after the other for a total of 30 minutes. One activity may last longer than others. Discuss your results of the triathlon in class.

Time: 30 minutes

Please return by _____.

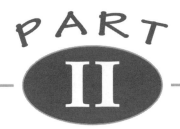
Lesson Elements

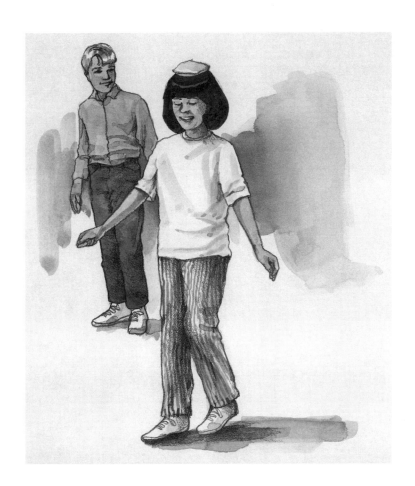

CHAPTER 10

Stretching Routines

Routine 1

For use on the playground (outside) where students cannot lie on the ground (see fig. 10.1).

A. Neck

Keeping shoulders back and spine straight, slowly roll the head to the left shoulder, straighten; then roll toward right shoulder, straighten. Repeat five times. *Do not* roll head in a fast, circular manner or roll head backward.

B. Back stretch (shoulder and upper arm)

Lift right arm and reach behind head and down the spine. With left hand, push down on right elbow and hold. Reverse arm positions and repeat.

C. Side bender (side of body)

Stretch left arm overhead to right. Bend to right at waist, reaching as far to right as possible with the left arm; reach as far as possible to the left with right arm, hold. Repeat on opposite side.

D. Knee pumps (back of upper leg)

While standing, hold the left leg behind the knee and draw it toward your chest. Hold 10 seconds, switch legs, and repeat three times.

E. Heel and toe raise (calf muscles)

Stand with feet close together, hands on hips. Raise up on toes, then heels. Repeat three times.

F. Hip circles (stomach and low back)

Keeping feet and head still, slowly rotate the hips in a sweeping circular motion to loosen the midsection. Repeat 10 times and change direction.

Routine 2

For use inside a gym, multipurpose room, or classroom where students can lie on the floor to stretch (see fig. 10.2).

A. Neck

Keeping shoulders back and spine straight, slowly roll the head to the left shoulder, straighten; then roll toward right shoulder, straighten. Repeat five times. *Do not* roll head in fast, circular manner or roll head backward.

B. Knee to nose touch (legs and stomach)

In an all fours position, lift the knee to touch the nose. Move the leg back so the leg does not lift higher than the hips, and the neck and lower back are not hyperextended.

C. Shin stretcher (shins)

Kneel on both knees, turn to right and press down on right ankle with right hand and hold. Keep hips thrust forward to avoid hyperflexing knees. *Do not* sit on heels. Repeat on left side.

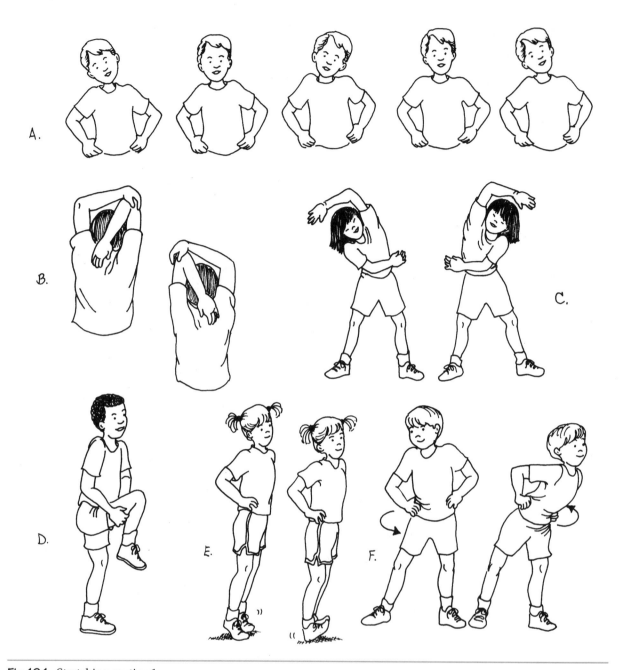

Fig. 10.1. Stretching routine 1

D. Single leg tuck (back of leg and lower back)

Sit on floor with left leg straight. Tuck right foot against left thigh. Lower chest toward left knee. Repeat with right leg.

E. Low-back stretch (low-back muscles)

Lie on back, and tuck knees to chest.

Routine 3

For use inside a gym, multipurpose room, or classroom where students can lie on the floor to stretch (see fig. 10.3).

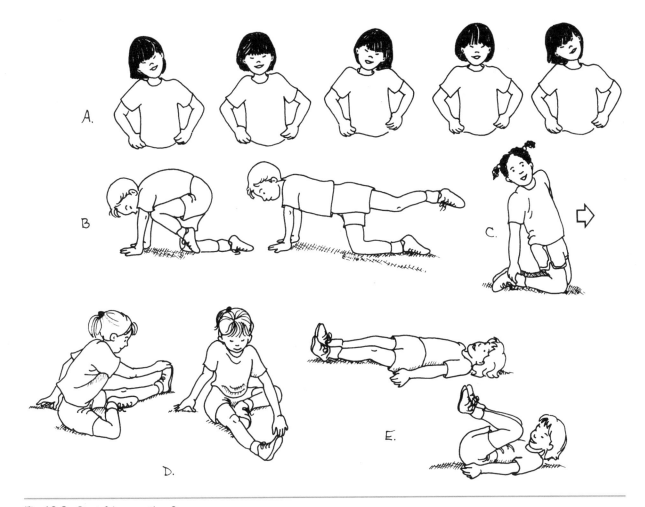

Fig. 10.2. Stretching routine 2

A. Sitting stretch (inside of thighs)

Sit with soles of feet together, place hands on knees or ankles, and lean forearms against knees. Resist while attempting to raise knees.

B. Behind neck grasp (back of arms)

Lift right arm and reach behind head and down the spine. With the left hand, reach behind back and grasp the right hand. Reverse hands.

C. One leg stretcher (lower back and back of legs)

Stand with one foot on a bench, keeping both legs straight. Press down on bench with the heel for several seconds; then relax and bend the trunk forward, trying to touch the head to the knee. Hold for a few seconds. Return to starting position and repeat with opposite leg. As flexibility increases, the arms can pull the chest toward the legs. Do not lock knee.

D. Arm stretcher (arms and chest)

Cross arms and turn palms of hands together. Raise arms overhead behind ears. Extend at the elbows. Reach as high as possible.

E. Trunk twister (trunk muscles)

Sit with right leg extended, left leg bent and crossed over right knee. Place right arm on the left side of the left leg, and push against that leg while turning the trunk as far as possible to the left. Place left hand on floor behind buttocks. Reverse position and repeat on opposite side.

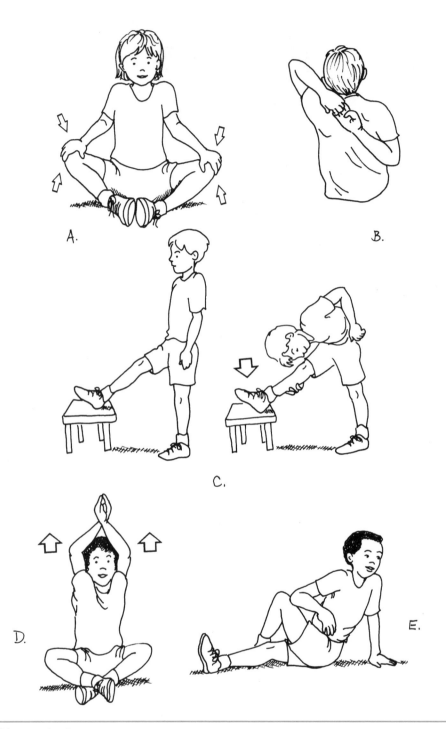

Fig. 10.3. Stretching routine 3

Warm-Up Activities

Select warm-ups that allow easy transition to the main activity of lesson. For example, the first warm-up would be ideal if the main focus of the lesson is jumping rope. The equipment is already available.

Jump rope and stretch

Each student has a jump rope and slowly starts jumping. On signal, the student performs a stretch using the jump rope. An example would be to fold the rope in half and hold it overhead while bending from side to side and to the toes.

Ready, draw!

With partners, each player starts with hands behind their backs. On "Draw," the players show either one or two fingers. If the players show different numbers, they do 10 repetitions of an exercise, for example, jumping jacks. If they show the same numbers, they do nothing and "Draw" again.

Line jump

Students stand next to a line on the playground or in the gym. They jump from side to side without touching the line for 30 seconds. How many times did you cross the line? Try again to see if your score improves on a second attempt.

Triangle tag

In groups of four, two students face each other and hold hands. The other two stand on either side of the students holding hands. One person is "it" and is chased by the other. The two holding hands act as a shield to the one being chased.

Fifteen-second gusto

15 seconds of jumping jacks
15 seconds of sit-ups
15 seconds of line jumps
15 seconds of jogging on the spot, bringing knees up high
15 seconds of modified push-ups

Court line tag

Students play on a basketball court, scattering anywhere on lines. All tags are made below the shoulder with Nerf balls. The two taggers, who tag with Nerf balls, start in the center. During game, players must stay on lines. If tagged, a player takes Nerf ball and immediately becomes a new tagger. Original tagger cannot be immediately tagged.

Kanga ball

In groups of three, two partners face each other and roll a ball back and forth. The third child stands between the pair and jumps over the ball, but turns to keep an eye on it. Roll the ball slowly at first. The objective is not to hit the player in the middle, but to make the player jump. Players can kick the ball back and forth or sit with their legs spread and roll the ball. The jumper can ask the others to vary the speed or keep it the same, according to ability. You can use balls of different sizes, and children change roles after 45 seconds.

Cigarette pack

This game is like smoking cigarettes. The more you smoke, the more difficulty you have being active. Designate an area of gym or playground as playing area. Select one person to be the cigarette, who chases others and tags them. The tagged players hook elbows or join hands and continue chasing others. The "cigarette chain" grows and grows. As it does, it has more difficulty moving. Split into two after chain reaches six players.

Partner cruise

Begin the activity with the students walking in a scatter formation around the gym. On command, have each student find a partner to face and shake their hand. This person is designated their "Handshake" partner. Again, the students scatter throughout the gym. On command, they must find their Handshake partners and shake hands. They then find a second partner and create a different handshake. The activity continues with students finding different partners and doing a different action with each partner, such as Back to Back, High Five, Sole Shake, and so on. Between partners, students walk or jog.

Over and under

Students find a partner. One partner makes a bridge on the floor while the other moves over, under, and around the bridge. This continues until you give a signal to switch, which notifies them to change positions. Try different types of bridges and movements.

Crossover

Divide children into groups of three, two on one side of the gym and one on the other. The one student calls one of the two students over by saying, "Crossover, Crossover Johnny come over doing a slow jog." Children take turns calling and say a different movement each time.

Bear moves

Find your favorite stuffed teddy bear. Face the class with the teddy bear so all students can see the bear. Move the bear's body parts into stretches and students follow the bear's moves. Students enjoy focusing on the bear and its moves. Select a bear whose body parts move easily

Bean bag boogie

Each student has a bean bag placed on their head. Students move around the gym trying to keep the bean bag on their heads. If the student loses the bag, they freeze and another student has to come and pick it up for them.

Circle tag

Set up two concentric circles. Organize children into a large circle, with 10 feet between each child. With chalk, mark a circle for children to run around. Each child tries to tag the next child ahead in the circle. Tagged children move to an inside circle (marked in chalk) and run counter-clockwise trying to tag the person in front of them. Children who are tagged on the inside circle move to the outside circle, changing directions as they switch circles.

Listen and move

Give the following instructions as quickly as the children can complete the tasks: run 20 steps to the left, skip 10 steps forward, jump as high as you can 10 times, make 5 big arm circles, gallop 20 steps forward, hop on the left foot 5 times, hop on the right foot 5 times.

Cool-Down Activities

Select cool-downs that allow an easy transition. For example, if children are already in pairs, the Meeting and Parting cool-down may be appropriate.

Rhythm run

Students form pairs and jog side by side around a baseball diamond or basketball court. Instruct them to run so their left and right feet move in rhythm together. When they can do this in pairs, have them progress to groups of four. Encourage students to remind their running partner to use good running techniques:

- Use arms by swinging forward and backward with elbows bent.
- Keep head still and upright.
- Heel hits ground first.
- Legs and feet swing and land straight ahead.

Slowly, change from jogging to walking.

Slo-mo skip

Set up four cones in square (40 × 40 yards). Students start by skipping one circuit at a fast rate, and each circuit thereafter slow down a little until they are in slo-mo.

Leader cruise

Use the rectangular area marked by cones. Line up the class in two lines side by side. The entire class starts with a jog. The two students at the end jog to the front. As soon as the new leaders are in front, the next two jog to the front. Progressively, the lines slow down until they are walking.

Raggedy Ann (or Andy)

Use the following poem:

Raggedy Ann is my best friend,
She's so floppy, just see her bend,
First at the waist, then at the knee,
Her arms are swinging wide and free,
Her head rolls like a rubber ball,
She hasn't any bones at all.
Raggedy Ann is stuffed with rags,
That's why her body wigs and wags.

Students can use the words of the poem to move their bodies in a relaxing way as they walk.

Meeting and parting

Start with a partner in a specific place in the playing area. Jog side by side, moving apart from each other (for 10–20 yards) and then meeting again. Maintain eye contact with each other. Watch for others. Start by jogging; then slowly reduce pace to a fast walk, then a slower walk.

Body shapes

Students make their bodies into specific shapes, for example, narrow, round, twisted, crooked, small, flat, pointed, wide, curled. Start by having children move quickly from one shape to another; then slow down, asking children to move as slowly as possible.

Statue run

Students run and on a signal assume a statue pose a few seconds before jogging again.

Team train

In groups of four or five, students stand in single file, holding on to the waist of the person in front. The leader moves the train around the play area. Change leaders. Trains begin to move slower as the cool-down continues.

Agility run

In playing area put out cones, and students have to weave in and out of them, careful not to collide with each other. Emphasize weaving patterns. Slow down as cool-down continues.

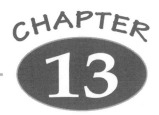
Exercises

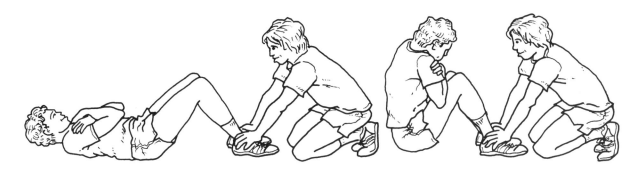

Sit-ups. Lie on back with knees bent (12–18 inch gap between feet and buttocks) and arms across chest. Lift upper body toward knees until arms touch thighs and lower until midback touches floor.

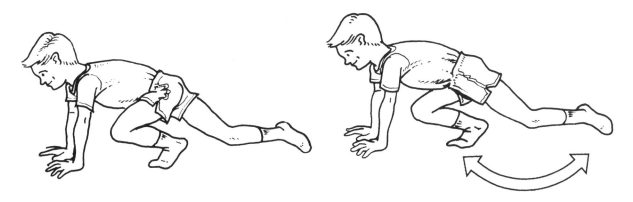

Mountain climbers. In front support position, bring the right knee up under chest and extend the left leg backward. Quickly switch leg positions, keeping a rhythmic movement pattern.

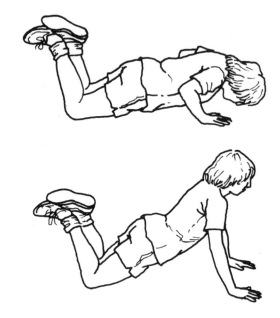

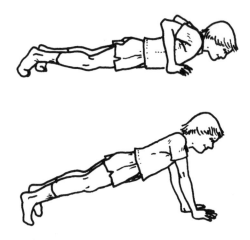

Push-ups.   Lie on stomach with chest touching floor and feet together. Hands are under the shoulders. Push and raise body by extending arms. Raise body in straight line, not allowing back to sway. Lower body until chin touches ground.

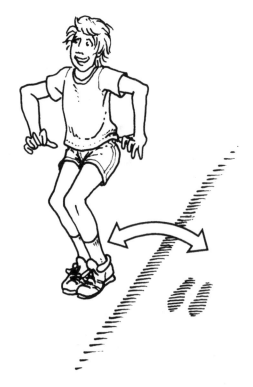

Modified push-ups.   Do as regular push-ups, only push up from knees, not feet.

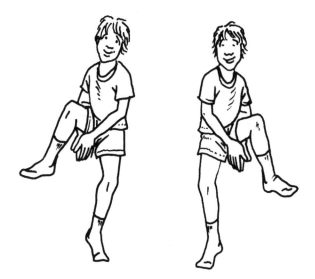

Clappers.   Hop on left foot, kick the right leg up, and clap your hands under the right leg. Hop on the right foot, kick the left leg up, and clap your hands under it. Land on the ball of the foot each time.

Skier.   With both feet together, jump from side to side over a line or jump rope.

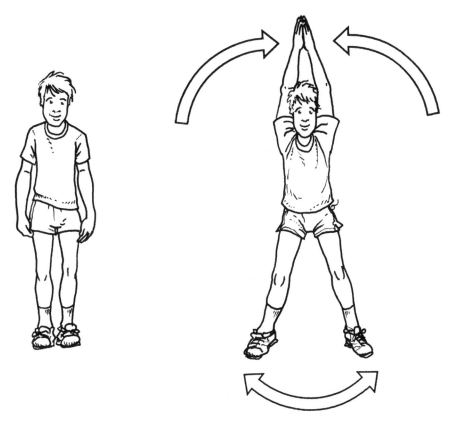

Jumping jacks. Stand with arms by sides. Simultaneously raise arms above head and move legs shoulder-width apart. Then bring arms to sides and feet together.

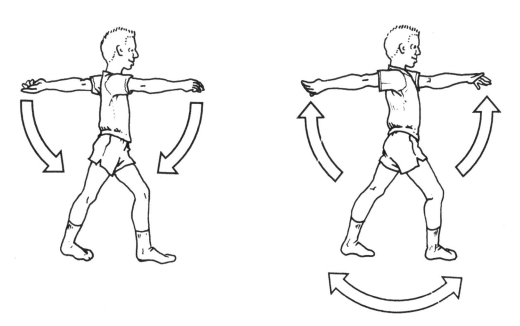

Cross-country skier. Stand with one foot in front and one foot behind body. The opposite arm is also in front of the body. Jump and change positions of feet and arms.

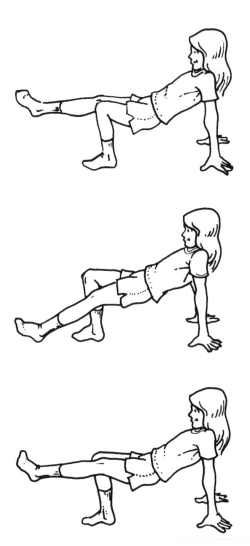

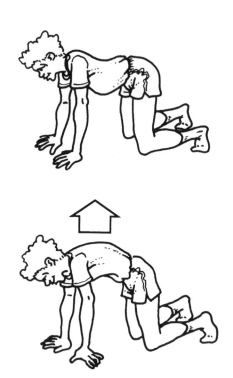

Bridge back.   On hands and knees in a crawling position, contract abdominal muscles and arch back as high as possible. Return to starting position.

Crab legs.   Support weight on hands and feet. Alternatively kick legs out away from body. Each kick counts as one repetition.

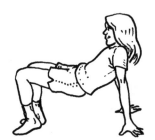

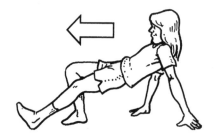

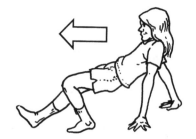

Crab walker.   From sitting position, push body off the ground and support weight on hands and feet. Move body forward three steps and backward three steps.

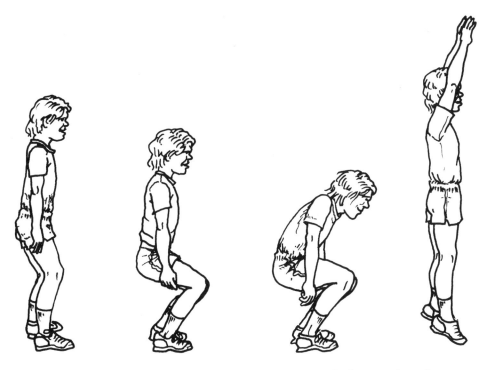

Jack-in-the-box.   Squat down low and pretend you are hiding in a box. Spring up reaching as high as you can. Return to starting position.

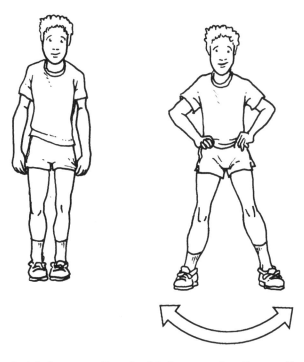

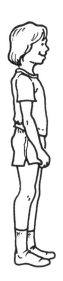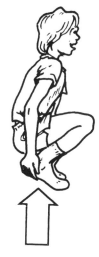

Heel touches.   Stand in an upright position with feet shoulder-width apart and arms fully extended at the sides. Jump vertically and touch the heels with the hands as the knees move to the chest.

Stride jumps.   Stand with feet together. Jump off ground so feet are spread three feet apart. Return to starting position.

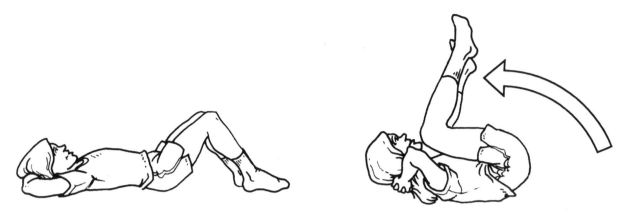

Reverse sit-ups.   Lie on back with legs together and knees bent. Bend at the waist and bring knees to chest. Lower legs to starting position.

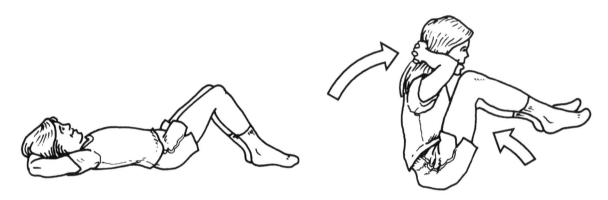

Crunches.   Lie on back with legs together and legs and knees bent, forming a 90-degree angle. Hands are behind head. Bring knees and elbows together, directly over waist area. Return to starting position.

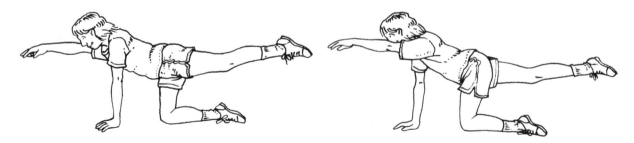

Cross body lift.   Assume an all fours position with your hands on the floor directly under your shoulders. In this position, raise one arm and the opposite leg simultaneously until they are slightly higher than your back. Then lower both simultaneously. Repeat this action with the opposite arm and leg in alternating fashion.

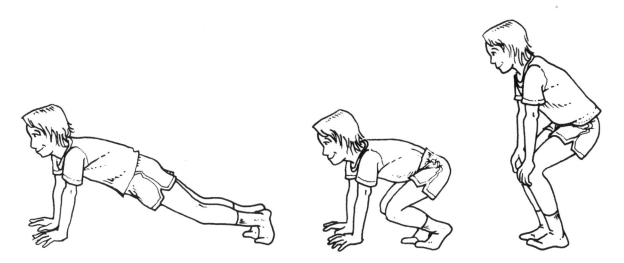

Squat thrusts.   In push-up position quickly move legs toward hands and jump high into the air.

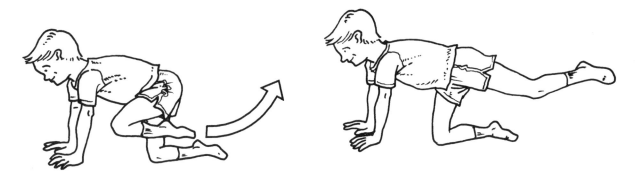

Leg extensions.   On all fours with legs square and right knee bent, raise right leg to side. Extend your leg forward and backward, parallel to the floor, then lower to the ground. Move legs only and keep upper body still. Change legs.

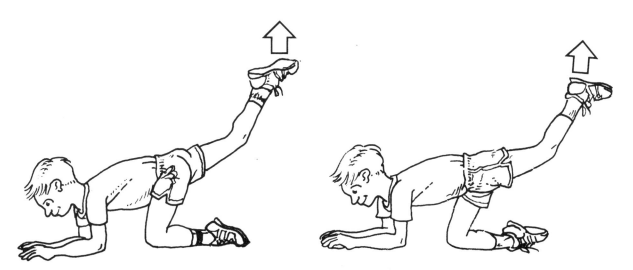

Skyscrapers.   Kneel on all fours. Lower weight to forearms and tighten abdominal muscles. Raise bent leg behind and push it to the ceiling. Flex and point the foot.

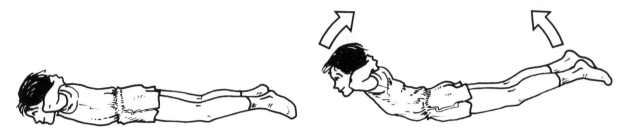

Chest raises.   Lie on stomach with feet together and hands clasped behind head. Raise head and chest away from ground and slowly lower to starting position.

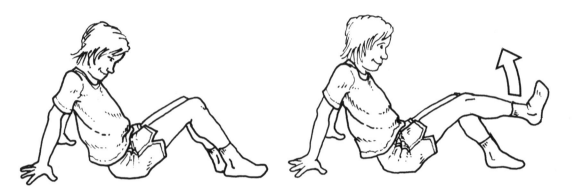

Thigh lifts.   Begin in the half-hook, half-long sit position. Raise and lower the extended leg. Change leg and raise.

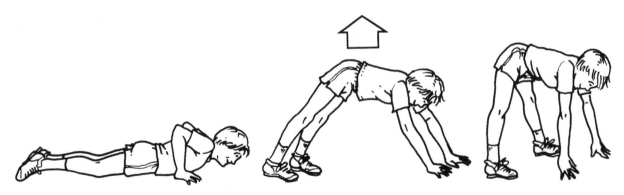

Inchworm.   Lie on stomach. Keep hands still and take small steps forward toward your hands. Then move feet back away from hands to the lying position.

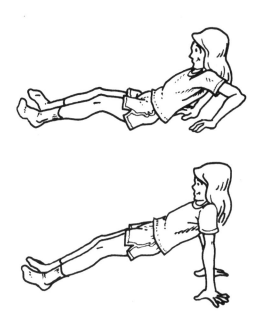

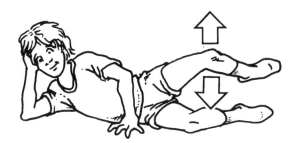

Side leg raises.   Lie on your right side with your head resting on your right hand and your left hand flat on the mat in front of you for support. Raise your upper leg. Repeat, changing sides.

Reverse push-ups.   In back support position, bend elbows to slowly lower body to the floor. Straighten elbows to raise body away from floor.

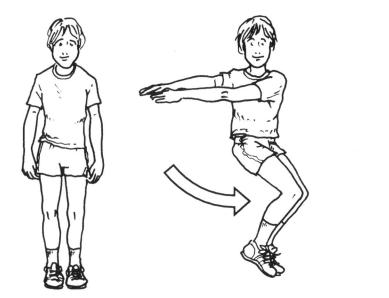

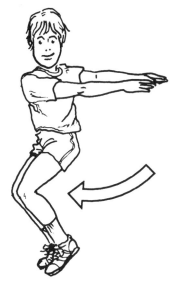

Jump twisters.   Stand with feet together, knees slightly bent. Thrust both arms to right while moving legs (from waist) to the left. Reverse action with arms moving to the left and legs to the right.

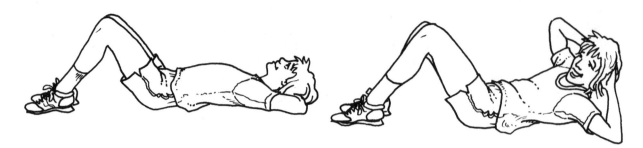

Obliques. Lie on back with knees bent, feet on floor with hands held lightly behind head. Lift shoulder and upper torso off the floor twisting one elbow toward opposite knee. Do not pull head and neck with hands. Return to starting position and repeat on other side. Press spine to floor so hips do not roll.

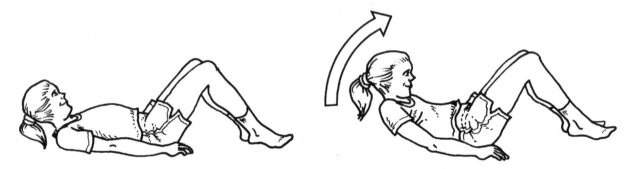

Curl-ups. Lie on back with knees at a 90-degree angle and arms extended by side. Lift head until upper back is raised from floor and the chin touches the chest. Return to floor.

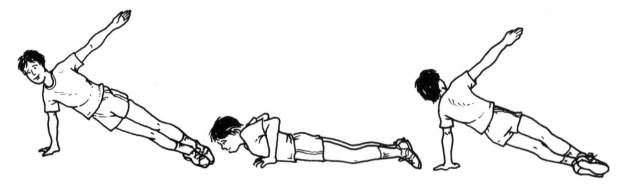

Side standers. Lie on stomach with chest touching floor. Raise body in push-up fashion and rotate body so you support weight on right hand and foot. Return to starting position and support weight on left hand and foot.

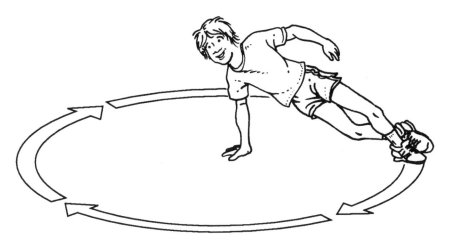

Coffee grinder.   Pivot on a supporting hand. Work feet around hand,
making a complete circle while keeping the body straight.

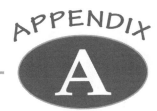

APPENDIX

A

Physical Fitness Testing

Physical fitness testing has traditionally been a part of physical education. We believe this should continue, but with the following concepts clearly in mind:

- Teach children to test themselves. Children who learn to test themselves will know their current fitness levels and develop skills to use in later life.
- Self-evaluation, rather than comparison to others is important. Heredity, maturity, and age have much to do with fitness performance. Use test results to help students plan personal fitness programs.
- Explain why fitness testing is important. Reaching acceptable health fitness standards provided by programs, helping children identify their own strengths and weaknesses, and allowing children to monitor their improvement are all good reasons for physical fitness testing.
- If you are going to use awards, clearly explain the procedure for receiving awards. Use an incentive program that rewards participation and effort.

The following physical fitness test programs are available:

Physical Best
American Alliance for Health, Physical Education, Recreation and Dance
1900 Association Drive
Reston, VA 22091.

President's Challenge
President's Council on Physical Fitness and Sports
450 Fifth Street NW, Room 7103
Washington, DC 20001.

Physical Fitness Program
Amateur Athletic Union
Poplars Building
Bloomington, IN 47405.

Fitnessgram
Institute for Aerobic Fitness Research
12330 Preston Road
Dallas, TX 74230
1-800-635-7050.

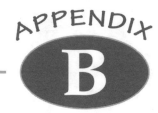

Parent Letter

You may use this sample letter as a guide for informing parents of the program and soliciting their involvement, or you may want to develop your own format. The goal for the program is to improve attitudes toward fitness in both students and parents, and to increase communication between the home and school.

Dear Parents:

Your child will be participating in a new physical fitness program soon. The name of the program is Health-Related Fitness. It will begin on (date) and run approximately _____ weeks.

In this program, we will explore a variety of topics related to health, physical fitness, and nutrition. We will emphasize establishing healthy habits that will last a lifetime. Students will learn how to assess their individual fitness level based on the knowledge they gain in this program and will be able to design their personal fitness program. They will learn how to maintain a healthy level of physical fitness. Also, they will learn about heart-healthy nutrition and how to improve their eating habits.

Your child will be involved in a wide range of fitness and nutrition activities. The weekly schedule is three days of physical activity and two days of classroom instruction. Students will be expected to perform only at their own level. Our goal is to help each student strive for and recognize individual gains in his or her fitness level.

If you have questions or would like further information about this program, please contact me by phone or letter. You will be receiving information about Family Fitness activities. We hope you will be able to participate and enjoy the fun with your children. We hope you can give support and encouragement to your child for continued improvement in health and fitness.

Please call me if you have any questions.

Sincerely,

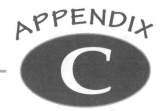

APPENDIX
C

Additional Resources

Bennett, J.P., and A. Kamiya. 1986. *Fitness and fun for everyone.* Durham, NC: Great Activities.

Cames, C. 1983. *Awesome elementary school physical education activities.* Carmichael, CA: Education.

Corbin, C.B., and R.P. Pangrazi. 1990. *Teaching strategies for improving youth fitness.* Dallas: Institute for Aerobics Research.

Foster, E.R., K. Hartinger, and K.A. Smith. 1992. *Fitness fun.* Champaign, IL: Human Kinetics.

Hopper, C. 1988. *The sports confident child.* New York: Pantheon Books.

Landy, J.M., and M.L. Landy. 1992. *Ready-to-use P.E. activities for grades K-2.* West Nyack, NY: Parker.

Pangrazi, R.P., and V.P. Dauer. 1992. *Dynamic physical education for elementary school children.* New York: Macmillan.

Petray, C.K., and S.L. Blazer. 1987. *Health-related physical fitness.* Edina, MN: Burgess.

Stillwell, J.L., and J.R. Stockard. 1988. *More fitness activities for children.* Durham, NC: Great Activities.

Index

About the Authors

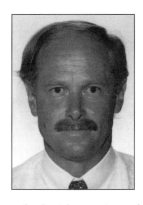

Chris Hopper, PhD, is department chair and professor of physical education at Humboldt State University in Arcata, California.

Hopper brings a variety of experiences in physical education to his writing. Since 1976 he has taught physical education at the elementary through college level. He also has consulted with a variety of organizations, including the United States Department of Education, the Boys Clubs of America, and the American Sport Education Program. Throughout his career he has coached both youth and collegiate soccer, serving as head coach of men's soccer at Humboldt State University.

In 1982 Hopper earned his PhD in physical education from the University of Oregon. Much of his research has focused on improving children's physical fitness and nutrition. He has published numerous articles in the *Journal of Physical Education, Recreation and Dance; Scholastic Coach; Adapted Physical Activity Quarterly;* and the *Research Quarterly for Exercise and Sport.* He is coauthor of *Coaching Soccer Effectively* and author of *The Sports-Confident Child.*

Hopper is a member of the American Alliance for Health, Physical Education, Recreation and Dance, the National Consortium on Physical Education and Recreation for Individuals With Disabilities; and the American Council on Rural Special Education.

Hopper, who lives in Ferndale, California, with his wife, Renee, and their three children, enjoys soccer, golf, and waterskiing.

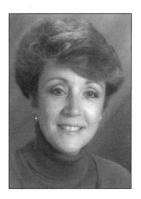

Kathy D. Munoz, EdD, is assistant professor in the Department of Health and Physical Education at Humboldt State University.

Munoz has a master's in food and nutrition from Oregon State University and an EdD in education and curriculum design from the University of Southern California. As a registered dietitian and home economics teacher, she has taught nutrition to a wide variety of ages and backgrounds, including secondary, community college, and university students. She also worked with students, athletes, and community members as a counselor at the Eating Disorder Clinic in Humboldt.

In 1989 Munoz won the Meritorious Performance and Professional Promise Award from Humboldt State for teaching nutrition. She is advisor to the Youth Education Services (YES) Nutrition for Kids program, a role she filled also for the Student Home Economics Association.

A member of the American Dietetic Association, American College of Nutrition, and the Society for Nutrition Education, Munoz lives in Fortuna, California, with her husband, Richard, and their three children. She pursues outdoor sports, reading, and traveling in her spare time.

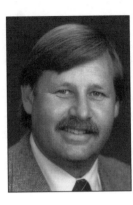

Bruce Fisher has received several honors for teaching excellence, including 1991 California Teacher of the Year, 1991 Professional Best Award, and the ABC-TV Favorite Teacher Award. A classroom teacher since 1975, he has created meaningful activities and lessons to teach fitness and nutrition to students at all grade levels.

As a member of the California State Department of Education's Health and Physical Education committee since 1991, Fisher helped design and develop the health and physical education frameworks for California. He has served on educational and curriculum development committees throughout his career, including the Family Wellness Project, and he also has presented at education conferences across the country.

In 1991 Fisher wrote the feature article for *Learning Magazine* on health and nutrition. Now with the Jet Propulsion Lab, Johns Hopkins University, and San Diego State University, he is writing the curriculum for NASA's KidSat/Project YES.

Fisher lives in Fieldbrook, California, with his wife, Mindi, and their daughter, Jenny. His hobbies include aviation, aerospace, astronomy, and photography.

Integrate health and fitness lessons into your curriculum with these ready-to-use activities

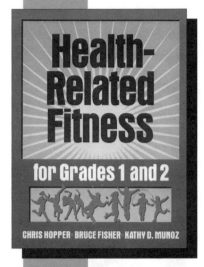

1996 • Paper • 128 pp
Item BHOP0498
ISBN 0-87322-498-1
$16.00 ($23.95 Canadian)

1996 • Paper • 136 pp
Item BHOP0499
ISBN 0-87322-499-X
$16.00 ($23.95 Canadian)

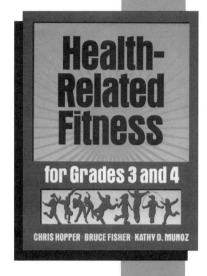

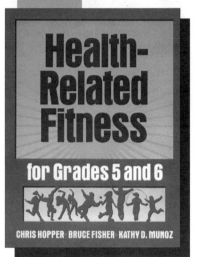

1996 • Paper • Approx 160 pp
Item BHOP0480
ISBN 0-88011-480-0
$18.00 ($26.95 Canadian)

Each *Health-Related Fitness* book provides 45 grade-appropriate, cross-curricular lessons and activities in physical fitness and nutrition. The classroom-tested programs in each book provide nine weeks of plans for five 30-minute, ready-to-use lessons.

This unique, hands-on curriculum includes homework assignments with family activities, cooperative learning experiences, cross-curricular activities to stimulate critical thinking skills, reproducible handouts, easy-to-understand adaptable scripts, activities based on state and national health standards, and lessons that require either no equipment or simple materials readily available. **Part I** of each book outlines lessons on cardiovascular fitness, strength, endurance, flexibility, and nutrition to help you prepare students for a healthy lifestyle. **Part II** describes the different kinds of elements you should teach in each lesson, including stretches, warm-ups, cool-downs, and exercises.

Special Package Price
All 3 *Health-Related Fitness* books • Item BHOP0668 • ISBN 0-88011-668-4
$43.00 ($64.50 Canadian)

Human Kinetics
The Information Leader in Physical Activity
http://www.humankinetics.com/

Prices are subject to change.

To place your order, U.S. customers **call TOLL FREE 1-800-747-4457**.
Customers outside the U.S. place your order using the appropriate
telephone number/address shown in the front of this book.

M8133-IN
89